# Ancient Fragments: Containing What Remains of the Writings of Sanchoniatho, Berossus, Abydenus, Megasthenes, and Manetho

Isaac Preston Cory

Frontier Model Bibliophile

**Ancient Fragments: Containing What Remains of the Writings of Sanchoniatho, Berossus, Abydenus, Megasthenes, and Manetho**

A Frontier Model Bibliophile facsimile edition.

Published by Big Five Killer (Nimble Books LLC),
Ann Arbor, Michigan, USA.



ISBN 9798259502451

BISAC: HIS002000 (HISTORY / Ancient / General)

---

*AI authorship disclosure.* Frontier Model Bibliophile is itself a frontier large-language model, openly so. It selects, frames, and produces the editorial apparatus of every volume in this imprint — in compliance with EU AI Act Article 50. The original text reproduced in this volume is a human-authored work in the public domain; see the Bibliographic Note for source details.

# Note on the Edition

Ancient Fragments is a working compendium, not a treatise. What Isaac Preston Cory produced in 1828 is closer in spirit to a sourcebook than to a history: a single bound volume in which the surviving paragraphs of the lost native historians of the pre-classical Near East are assembled, set in their original Greek (or Latin) beside an English translation, and prefaced with the minimum of editorial scaffolding a reader requires to use them. The named authors are spectral presences in the surviving literature. Sanchoniatho of Phoenicia survives only inside Eusebius of Caesarea, whose Praeparatio Evangelica preserved excerpts from Philo of Byblos's lost Greek translation of an originally Phoenician work whose date is itself contested. Berossus, the Babylonian priest of Bel-Marduk who flourished under the early Seleucids, survives in scattered citations by Josephus, Eusebius, and the ninth-century chronographer George Syncellus, themselves working from the now-lost epitome of Alexander Polyhistor. Manetho of Egypt comes down to us almost entirely through later chronographers, his dynastic lists transmitted second- and third-hand through Africanus, Eusebius, and Syncellus. Megasthenes on India is fragmentary. To these Cory adds the Hermetic creed, the Old Chronicle, the Laterculus of Eratosthenes, the Tyrian Annals, the Chaldean Oracles attributed to Zoroaster, and the Periplus of Hanno the Carthaginian. The animating premise is that these scraps, taken together, are nearly all that survives of the literatures of Assyria, Babylon, Persia, Egypt, Phoenicia, Tyre, and Carthage in their own voices, and that they accordingly deserve to be gathered, classified, and made available as a single working corpus.

The book came out of a particular intellectual moment. Cory was a Cambridge man — a fellow of Caius — writing in the tradition of Jacob Bryant's three-volume A New System; or, An Analysis of Ancient Mythology (1774-76) and George Stanley Faber's three-volume Origin of Pagan Idolatry (1816), both of which appear by name in the preface as the authorities for the larger interpretive frame. The project of that tradition assumed that the heathen records, properly arranged, would corroborate the early chapters of Genesis. The flood narrative attributed to Berossus, the antediluvian genealogies in Sanchoniatho, the long Egyptian dynasty lists in the Laterculus and in Manetho — all are read by Cory and his contemporaries as parallel testimony to events that the Hebrew scriptures recorded canonically, and as evidence that a single primordial human history lay behind the dispersed pagan theogonies. This is the pre-Assyriological frame: the cuneiform tablets had not yet been read, the Egyptian hieroglyphic inscriptions were only beginning to yield to Champollion's key, and the comparative method available to a London antiquary in 1828 was textual, etymological, and Biblical rather than archaeological.

What the present-day reader gets from the book is twofold. First, the actual texts. Whatever has been done with these fragments since — and Burstein on Berossus, Verbrugghe and Wickersham on Berossus and Manetho together, Attridge and Oden on the Eusebian Sanchoniathon transmission, and others have re-edited them under modern scholarly standards — Cory was the first to put them all in one accessible English volume. The Greek faces the translation column by column; the source citation (Eusebius Praeparatio Evangelica, Syncellus Chronographia, Josephus Contra Apionem) is supplied at every fragment, so a reader can in principle move from the page to the original transmitting work and check the context. Second, the book offers a window into how educated Britons in the 1820s understood the deep past before the great decipherments rewrote everything. The interpretive moves in Cory's prefatory remarks — the suggestion that Agrus the Phoenician husbandman corresponds to Noah, that Misor corresponds to the Biblical Mizraim, that the Greeks borrowed and allegorized originally historical Phoenician memories — are not eccentric. They are the working consensus of the British Biblical-antiquarian school as it stood on the eve of its replacement.

The method of this edition is reprint, not revision. The 1828 first edition is reproduced as Cory and his printer at William Pickering of Chancery Lane set it: the parallel Greek-English columns, the chapter introductions, the running citations to the transmitting authors, and the index. No emendation has been made to Cory's text, his Greek setting, his transliterations, or his identifications. The editorial apparatus that this Frontier Model Bibliophile edition supplies — the present note, the historical context, the about-the-author piece, and the annotated bibliography of works that transmit, supersede, or extend Cory's collection — is supplied separately. The facsimile and the apparatus are distinct; the reader can ignore the apparatus and have a clean Cory.

The experience this edition transmits is the moment of opening a quarto in 1828 and finding, side by side on the page, the Greek of Eusebius and an English sentence reporting that a god in Phoenicia was once called Agrus the husbandman.

— *Frontier Model Bibliophile*

# Source Note

Source: Internet Archive identifier `ancientfragments00coryuoft`, scanned from Internet Archive partner library. The interior of this Frontier Model Bibliophile edition is the unaltered source PDF, with FMB's front and back matter added.

Read Cory inside the frame of 1828, not 2026. He writes before the decipherment of cuneiform (Rawlinson's mature publications come in the 1850s) and before the full publication of Champollion's hieroglyphic system. The Babylonian and Egyptian sources he can use are entirely the Greek and Latin secondary citations. He also writes inside a tradition — Bryant, Faber, later Higgins — that treats the Genesis flood and the dispersion at Babel as historical events to which the pagan fragments offer corroborative testimony. Etymological identifications in the preface (Misor = Mizraim, Agrus = Noah, Chna = Canaan) reflect that program. They are the live scholarship of his decade and they should be read as such, not silently corrected. Cory's vocabulary — Phoenician, Chaldaean, Egyptian as the standing categories; the Bible as the master timeline against which everything else is checked — is the standard frame of the British Biblical antiquarian tradition. Modern scholarship has revised most of his identifications and replaced his transmitting sources with critical editions. The value of the volume is documentary: it shows what the textual record looked like, and what it was thought to mean, before the spade and the decipherer arrived.

# Bibliographic Note

*Ancient Fragments: Containing What Remains of the Writings of Sanchoniatho, Berossus, Abydenus, Megasthenes, and Manetho* by Isaac Preston Cory.

London: William Pickering, 1828 (first edition).

Reproduced facsimile total: 167 pages of source content, in addition to this edition's front and back matter.

# About the Author

Isaac Preston Cory was born in 1802 and died in 1842, a working life of barely two decades that nevertheless produced one of the standard reference volumes of pre-Assyriological Near Eastern scholarship. He was educated at Caius College, Cambridge, where he held a fellowship — the title page of Ancient Fragments identifies him as Fellow of Caius. His intellectual formation belonged to the late Georgian Cambridge tradition that combined classical learning with antiquarian and Biblical inquiry, and he wrote inside the lineage of Jacob Bryant and George Stanley Faber, both of whom he names in his preface as the authorities to whom he defers for the larger interpretive framework.

Ancient Fragments first appeared in 1828, when Cory was twenty-six. A second, expanded edition followed in 1832, adding among other things a fragment from the Indian Laws of Manu and additional material on Persian and Egyptian sources. Cory also published The Mythological Inquiry into the Recondite Theology of the Heathens (1833) and A Practical Treatise on Accounts (1839), the latter reflecting a quite different vein of activity. His Inquiry pursued the comparative-mythology project of his Bryantian predecessors, attempting to demonstrate that the pagan theogonies preserved, in disguised form, the same primordial revelation recorded in Genesis.

What shaped Cory's perspective was the conjunction of three things: a Cambridge classical training that gave him fluent Greek and the philological habits of textual collation; the still-dominant British antiquarian tradition that treated the early chapters of Genesis as a historical document whose substance was corroborated by pagan testimony; and the historical accident of working before the great decipherments. Had he lived another decade he would have seen Rawlinson's Behistun work begin to circulate; had he lived two more he would have seen Akkadian read. He did not. Ancient Fragments accordingly captures the state of the field on the eve of its transformation.

Cory died in 1842 at the age of forty. His legacy is the book reprinted here: the standard English collection of the pre-classical Near Eastern fragments for the better part of the nineteenth century, drawn on by every comparative mythologist of the period and reprinted in expanded form by E. Richmond Hodges in 1876.

# Public-Domain Statement

# How You Can Train On This Book

Cory's *Ancient Fragments* is, before anything else, a manual for a specific intellectual skill: reading-through-fragments. The book gathers what survives of Sanchoniatho, Berossus, Abydenus, Megasthenes, Manetho, the Hermetic books, the Old Chronicle, Eratosthenes' Laterculus of the kings of Thebes, the Tyrian Annals of Dius and Menander, the Oracles of Zoroaster, and the Periplus of Hanno — not as a connected narrative, but as quotations preserved *inside* the surviving works of later writers (Eusebius, Syncellus, Josephus, Alexander Polyhistor, Africanus, Apollodorus, Iamblichus). Every one of these primary sources reaches us only because some other writer happened to quote them. The original scrolls of Berossus's *Babyloniaca* and Manetho's *Aegyptiaca* are gone. The fragments are all that is left, and Cory's job in 1828 was to collect them, set the Greek (and occasional Latin) on the verso, his English on the recto, and supply just enough commentary to let a reader find their footing. That two-column layout — ancient tongue beside modern — is itself a piece of pedagogy. You watch the translator work. You can see where Cory pushes a phrase one way and where he hedges. That habit of always keeping the source visible is the discipline the book trains, and 178 octavo pages turn out to be more than enough room to install it.

What is still entirely valid in 2026 is the *method* on display in Cory's prefatory essay. He treats fragmentary evidence the way a careful editor still treats it. He names the intermediary at the foot of every passage (*Euseb. Praep. Evan. lib. 9*; *Syncel. Chron. 28*; *Joseph. contr. App. lib. I. c. 17*). He separates the words that probably belong to the original author from those that probably belong to the translator or epitomator — his note on Sanchoniatho's strictures against the Greeks, which he attributes to Philo of Byblos rather than to Sanchoniatho himself, is exactly this move (preface, page vi). He is openly tentative about which dynastic king-list to trust where Africanus and Eusebius disagree, and explicit about why he is preferring Africanus (preface, page xvi). He marks his own conjectures as conjectures, and prints competing conjectures of his predecessors (Faber, Bryant, Bishop Cumberland) so that the reader can compare them. That is still the protocol of modern scholarly editions. The two reference editions a 2026 reader will be sent to — Stanley Burstein's *The Babyloniaca of Berossus* (Sources from the Ancient Near East, 1978) and Verbrugghe & Wickersham's *Berossos and Manetho, Introduced and Translated* (University of Michigan Press, 1996) — do the same job Cory does, only with another 170 years of cuneiform, hieroglyphic, and papyrological evidence to cross-check the quotations against. Read Cory side by side with Verbrugghe & Wickersham on the Berossus deluge fragment (the Xisuthrus story, around pages 22–31 in Cory) and you can see the method evolving in real time: the same Greek passage, the same chain of intermediaries, but a vastly enlarged comparative frame.

What the book offers a reader who is paying attention is a way of *seeing* sources that has applications well beyond the ancient Near East. Cory wrestles publicly with three problems that have not gone away. First, the chronology problem: how to align Berossus's regnal years (ten antediluvian kings, 120 *sari*, 432,000 years before the flood, page 28) with Manetho's dynastic lists, with the Old Chronicle, with Eratosthenes' thirty-eight Theban kings (pages 78–84), and with biblical chronology. Modern Assyriology and Egyptology no longer try to reconcile any of these with Genesis, but they do still try to reconcile Berossus's kings with the Sumerian King List recovered from cuneiform tablets in the late nineteenth and early twentieth centuries, and Manetho's dynasties with the archaeological record. The reconciliation is unfinished. Second, the authenticity problem: which fragments are real, which are Hellenistic forgery, which have been quietly Christianised in transmission. Cory excludes the Sibylline Oracles and the books of Enoch on exactly this ground (preface, pages ii–iii) — a judgement modern editors largely uphold. Third, the typological problem: when a heathen source seems to "confirm" a biblical episode (Berossus on the deluge, Abydenus on the Tower of Babel, Dius on Solomon's correspondence with Hiram of Tyre), how much of the consonance is genuine memory of a shared event, how much is the Greek translator unconsciously importing his own framework, and how much is the Christian intermediary nudging the text? Cory does not pretend to settle this. He shows you the levers.

There are also things in the volume that have *not* survived into 2026 practice and are worth recovering. One is the unembarrassed practice of printing the Greek opposite the English on every page. The cost was real: it doubled the typesetting bill and required compositors who could set Greek. The benefit was that a reader with even a few terms of Greek could check the translator in real time, and a reader with no Greek at all could at least see where a fragment broke off, where an editor had restored a word, where a key term was being rendered tendentiously. Modern academic editions in the Loeb Classical Library still do this; trade reprints almost never do. Cory's volume is a working demonstration of why the facing-page convention earns its keep. A second recoverable practice is Cory's habit of citing the intermediary, with chapter and section, at the end of every fragment. He never just gives you "Berossus says." He gives you "*Syncel. Chron. 28. — Euseb. Chron. 5. 8*" — which means: this passage of Berossus reaches you via Syncellus's *Chronicle* at page 28, and is also independently preserved in Eusebius's *Chronicon* at book 5, chapter 8. That double-citation is what lets a later scholar evaluate whether the two chains agree, and whether the variants between them are scribal slips or substantive differences. In an age of footnoteless trade nonfiction and link-rotted web citations, that is a habit worth re-importing.

This is exactly the skill a 2026 reader can usefully practise on fragments that are, in their own way, contemporary. Heraclitus survives only in citations by later authors — read Miroslav Marcovich's edition alongside Charles Kahn's *The Art and Thought of Heraclitus* (Cambridge, 1979) and the parallel with Cory's Sanchoniatho is exact: a doxographer's quotation, embedded in another writer's argument, has to be peeled out of that argument before it can mean anything in its own right. Sappho's poems, recovered from Egyptian papyrus scraps and from quotations in Athenaeus and the grammarians, are reconstructed the same way; Anne Carson's *If Not, Winter* (Knopf, 2002) prints the gaps as gaps, the way Cory marks where the Berossus extracts break off and where Eratosthenes' Theban list has a missing king-name (page 84, the thirty-sixth king, where the name simply does not survive). The lost films of the silent era survive as stills, posters, scenarios, and trade-press reviews; the *Treasures from American Film Archives* series from the National Film Preservation Foundation reads them with the same protocol. Even early jazz and blues recordings — where the only surviving evidence of a 1922 take might be a single 78 rpm side and a contemporaneous catalogue listing — are read fragment-style; Dust-to-Digital's reissue work in the last twenty years is essentially the Cory method applied to shellac. Cory is training a transferable eye.

The specific concrete experience the book makes available, and the one most worth trying, is a side-by-side reading. Pick the Berossus deluge fragment in Cory (the Xisuthrus narrative, pages 22–31, with the Greek of Syncellus and Eusebius on the verso and Cory's English on the recto). Read it slowly once in Cory alone. Note what he tells you about the chain of transmission — the fragment comes through Alexander Polyhistor, who is quoted by Eusebius, who is in turn quoted by Syncellus, three intermediaries before you reach the page. Note where Cory's footnotes flag a textual variant. Then open Verbrugghe & Wickersham, or Burstein 1978, on the same fragment. Notice three things. First, what Cory *had* (the Greek as preserved in the chain of Christian chronographers) is essentially what the modern editor has: the textual base has not changed much. Second, what has been added: cross-references to the cuneiform deluge narratives recovered from Nineveh in the 1870s — *Atra-Hasīs* and the eleventh tablet of *Gilgamesh* — which Cory could not have known about, since George Smith would not present his translation of the Gilgamesh flood tablet to the Society of Biblical Archaeology until December 1872, forty-four years after Cory's volume appeared. Third, what has been subtracted: Cory's harmonising commitment to read every heathen flood story as a corruption of Noah's flood is no longer in the modern apparatus; the modern editor reads Berossus as evidence for Mesopotamian flood traditions on their own terms. That triangulation —

what stayed, what was added, what was dropped — is the single most useful exercise this book supports. Do it once with the deluge fragment, and you will have a working model of how a primary source ages: which parts of a two-hundred-year-old scholarly edition remain load-bearing, which have been quietly retired, and which have been replaced by evidence the editor could not have imagined. After that, the same exercise works on Manetho's Shepherd Kings (Cory's translation of Josephus's quotation of Manetho on page xvii of the preface and in the body, against Donald Redford's *Egypt, Canaan, and Israel in Ancient Times*, Princeton, 1992), on the Sanchoniatho cosmogony (against the Ugaritic tablets recovered from Ras Shamra in 1929 and after, and edited in Mark Smith's *Ugaritic Narrative Poetry*, Scholars Press, 1997), on the Tyrian Annals of Menander on the invasion of Shalmaneser (pages 90–92, against the Assyrian royal inscriptions edited in the State Archives of Assyria series), or on the Periplus of Hanno (against the modern reconstructions of West African coastal geography in Aubrey Diller's *The Tradition of the Minor Greek Geographers*). One careful weekend with the deluge fragment is enough to install the habit; once installed, the habit applies to every fragmentary source you will ever read.

# Historical Context

Cory's Ancient Fragments came off William Pickering's press in 1828, a date that sits exactly on the hinge between two intellectual eras. The decipherment of Egyptian hieroglyphs had been announced by Jean-Francois Champollion in his Lettre a M. Dacier in 1822 and developed in the Precis du systeme hieroglyphique in 1824, but the full implications were not yet absorbed by British antiquarian writing. Cuneiform remained unread. Henry Rawlinson, who would copy the Behistun inscription in 1835 and publish his decipherment of Old Persian cuneiform later in the decade, was in 1828 an East India Company cadet barely arrived in Bombay. Akkadian would not be readable for another generation. What this meant for a London scholar of the ancient Near East in 1828 was simple: the sources were Greek and Latin, and any access to Phoenicia, Babylon, or pharaonic Egypt ran through Eusebius, Josephus, Syncellus, and the handful of classical authors who had quoted now-lost native historians.

The book also sits inside a still-living British tradition of Biblical antiquarianism. Jacob Bryant's three-volume A New System; or, An Analysis of Ancient Mythology had appeared in 1774-76 and remained a touchstone; George Stanley Faber's three-volume The Origin of Pagan Idolatry came out in 1816. Cory names both in his preface and works in their idiom. The program of that tradition was to read the pagan fragments as scattered echoes of the events recorded in Genesis — the creation, the flood, the dispersion at Babel — and to recover, through etymological and mythological comparison, a unified pre-Mosaic history of mankind. Godfrey Higgins's vast Anacalypsis, posthumously published in 1833 and 1836, would carry this method to its most expansive form, and would draw on Cory.

The wider scholarly weather of the late 1820s included the steady professionalization of classical philology in Germany — August Boeckh's Corpus Inscriptionum Graecarum began appearing in 1828 — and the early stirrings of what would become Orientalism as a university discipline. The Royal Asiatic Society had been founded in London in 1823. James Prinsep, who would decipher Brahmi and Kharosthi scripts in India, was a contemporary working toward a different kind of pre-classical recovery. Champollion himself died in 1832, four years after Cory's first edition; Cory's own second edition would appear in 1832 and add a Sanskrit fragment from the Laws of Manu.

Literary London at the moment of publication was reading Walter Scott's late novels and the early volumes of Thomas Babington Macaulay in the Edinburgh Review. The Reform Bill crisis was four years away. Pickering's imprint — which Cory's title-page bears — was at the time one of the most distinguished scholarly publishers in the city, known for the Diamond Classics and for handsome editions of English divines and antiquaries. To have Pickering on the title page in 1828 placed Ancient Fragments in serious company and signaled that the volume was aimed at the learned reader rather than the popular market.

THE

# ANCIENT FRAGMENTS;

CONTAINING

WHAT REMAINS OF THE WRITINGS OF

SANCHONIATHO, BEROSSUS, ABYDENUS,
MEGASTHENES, AND MANETHO.

ALSO

THE HERMETIC CREED, THE OLD CHRONICLE,
THE LATERCULUS OF ERATOSTHENES,
THE TYRIAN ANNALS,
THE ORACLES OF ZOROASTER,
AND THE PERIPLUS OF HANNO.

BY I. P. CORY, ESQ.
FELLOW OF CAIUS COLLEGE, CAMBRIDGE.

LONDON:
WILLIAM PICKERING.
MDCCCXXVIII.

# PREFACE.

IN presenting this collection of ANCIENT FRAGMENTS to the world, some explanation of what is comprehended under that title is not altogether unnecessary. We are accustomed to regard the Hebrew scriptures, and the Greek and Latin writings, as the only certain records of antiquity: yet there have been other languages, in which have been written the annals and the histories of other countries. Where then are those of Assyria and Babylon, of Persia and Egypt and Phœnicia, of Tyre and Carthage? Of the literature of all these mighty empires where are even the remains? It will, no doubt, tend to excite some reflections of a melancholy cast, to look on this small volume as an answer. That they are all contained in it, I should be unwilling to assert: yet, with some diligence and research, I have not been able to discover other fragments, which I could consider sufficiently authenticated, to increase its size.

It was my wish to have included in this collection all the fragments of the earlier Gentile world, which have reached us through the medium of the

Greek language. Of the early historians of Greece the names only of some have come down to us; whilst of others, such as Eupolemus and Histiæus, several very interesting fragments have escaped the general wreck. In the classic ages of their literature, the acquaintance of the Greek historians with antiquity is generally confined and obscure: nor was it till the publication of the Septuagint, that they turned their attention to the antiquities of their own and the surrounding nations: and for this reason we meet with more certain notices of ancient history in the later, than in the earlier times of Greece. To have drawn a line then, to have inserted the earlier writers to the exclusion of the later, would have been to omit the more valuable. To have reprinted the fragments of many authors, such as Nicolaus Damascenus, a writer of Damascus, of the Augustan age, would have introduced, with some matter worthy of attention, much of little interest. To have selected from them all, the passages relating to ancient times and foreign states, would have been a task as useless as laborious, and would have swelled the collection to a series of volumes. I have therefore excluded all native Greek historians—and every writer of the Augustan age and downwards—I have also omitted all fragments which bear about them the stamp of forgery, or are the productions of Hellenistic Jews; or of authors who have had access to the sacred Scriptures, and following the words throw no additional light upon the subjects: under one or other of which divisions may be classed the Antediluvian books of Enoch, the large fragments of Artapanus, the Sibylline Oracles, the correspondence of Solomon and Hiram king of Tyre, the tragedy of Ezekiel in which Moses figures as the hero, with several compositions of a similar description.

The contents then of this volume are Fragments which have been translated from foreign languages into Greek; or have been quoted or transcribed by Greeks from foreign authors; or have been written in the Greek language by foreigners who have had access to the archives of their own respective countries. They are arranged under the following heads: the Phœnician, the Chaldæan, the Egyptian, the Tyrian, the Persian, and the Carthaginian.

In the following review of these ancient writers, I have passed from themselves into a slight examination of their works: not with a view of entering at all into the details, but merely to call the attention to some few great landmarks, which stand prominently forth amidst what might otherwise be deemed a wild, pathless and interminable. For the most ample and satisfactory explanation of the whole, I must refer to the inimitable works of Mr. Faber and Bryant.

Under the first head is contained only the Phœnician Theology of Sanchoniatho, who is considered to be the most ancient writer of the heathen world. In what age he wrote is uncertain: but his history was composed in the Phœnician language, and its materials collected from the archives of the Phœnician cities. It was translated into Greek by Philo Byblius, and for the preservation of these fragments we are indebted to the care of Eusebius. I have deviated but little from the quaint translation of Bishop Cumberland, generally so far only as to render it more consonant with the text of Stephen, or to substitute more modern expressions for phrases become now almost obsolete.

The cosmogony is one of those jargons of Theology and Physics, which were refined by the later heathens into some resemblance of the sublimest mystery of the Christian faith. As the most ancient, it is the most valuable; and as it speaks more plainly than the rest, it affords a key to their interpretation.

The generations contain many very curious passages. They are the only well authenticated heathen account of the times before the flood.

In the first generation is an allusion to the fall: in the second Genus may be Cain: after which we lose the traces of similarity: at the fifth there is an interruption. But taking up the thread of inquiry, at the end of the first line, in Taautus or Thoyth, we may perhaps recognize Athothis, the second king of Egypt, the Hermes Trismegistus, who appears again as the adviser of Cronus. His predecessor Misor, corresponds then with Mizraïm, the first king of Egypt, the Menes and Mines of the dynasties. In the preceding generation is Amynus, Ammon, or Ham, the same with the Cronus, of what is supposed a different line. An ascent higher we find, Agrus, the husbandman, who was worshipped in Phœnicia as the greatest of the gods: he corresponds with Noah, the Ouranus of the other line, whose original name was Epigeus or Autochthon, a name of similar import with Agrus. There is also some slight appearance of identity between Hypsistus, the father of Autochthon or Ouranus, and Geïnus Autochthon, the father of Agrus.

The generations conclude with an intimation, that they contain the real history of those early times, stripped of the fictions and allegories with which it had been obscured by the son of Thabion, the first hierophant of Phœnicia. That such is the case we are assured by Philo Byblius, in the remarks on Sanchoniatho with which he prefaces his translation of the work. The passage also informs us that the history thus disguised was handed down to Isiris, the brother of Chna, the first Phœnician. Bishop Cumberland conjectures that this Isiris is the Osiris of the Egyptian worship, and with greater probability supposes him the same with Mizraïm, the son of Ham, who was the brother of Canaan. But he strangely wanders from the truth in his researches after the son of Thabion. If the legends were handed down to Isiris, the son of Ham, they must have been handed down by one of the predecessors of this Isiris, that is by Noah, or one of his own sons: Thabion is derived from Theba the Ark, and in the phraseology of Bryant is equivalent to the Arkite: it is a title of Noah: therefore the first hierophant of Phœnicia was a son of Noah, a predecessor of Mizraïm and Canaan, an inhabitant also of Phœnicia, in short was Ham himself. And it is some confirmation, indirect enough it must be owned, of the very prevalent belief in the apostacy of that patriarch.

This fragment is succeeded by a stricture on the propensity of the Greeks for allegory. Several of these strictures occur in the course of the extract. I have generally omitted them as they appear to be the words of Philo, the translator, and could never have been those of so early a writer as Sanchoniatho. But to exhibit the argument in the adverse light, it may be urged, that since these strictures on the Greeks occur, Sanchoniatho could not have written in such ancient times. Be that as it may, the passages have no connection with the history, and at any rate were not contained in the Phœnician records.

The last fragment, upon the mystical sacrifice of the Phœnicians, is so singular, that I cannot forbear inserting the conclusion of Bryant's dissertation on the subject. After having shewn that this is the only sacrifice among the ancients, which is termed *mystical;* and that Cronus, the personage who offers it was the chief deity of the Phœnicians; and moreover, that it could not relate to any previous transaction, he concludes thus:—

"The mystical sacrifice of the Phœnicians had these requisites, that a *prince was to offer it:* and *his only son was to be the victim:* and as I have shewn that this could not relate to any thing *prior;* let us consider what is said upon the subject, as *future,* and attend to the consequence. For if the sacrifice of the *Phœnicians* was a type of *another* to come; the nature of this last will be known from the representation, by which it was prefigured. According to this, *El,* the supreme deity, whose associates were the Elohim,* was in process of time to have a son, αγαπητον well-beloved: μονογενη, his only begotten: who was to be conceived (of ανωβρετ), as some render it, of *grace:* but according to my interpretation, of *the fountain of light.* He was to be called *Jeoud* whatever that name may relate to; and to be *offered up as a sacrifice to his father* λυτρον, by way of *satisfaction,* and *redemption,* τιμωρος δαιμοσι, *to atone for the sins of others,* and *avert the just vengeance of God;* αντι της παντων φθορας, to prevent universal corruption, and at the same time, *general ruin.* And it is farther remarkable; *he was to make*

* See page 11.

*the grand sacrifice* βασιλικῷ σχήματι κεκοσμημένος, *invested with the emblems of royalty.* These surely are very strong expressions: and the whole is an aggregate of circumstances highly significant, which *cannot be the result of chance.* All, that I have requested to be allowed me in the process of this recital, is this simple supposition, that *this mystical sacrifice was a type of something to come:* how truly it corresponds to that, which I imagine it alludes to, I submit to the reader's judgment. I think, it must be necessarily esteemed a most wonderful piece of history."

Sanchoniatho wrote also a history of the serpent. A single fragment of which is preserved by Eusebius.

The Chaldæan Fragments are chiefly from Berossus and Megasthenes.

Berossus, a Babylonian, flourished in the reign of Alexander, and lived some time at Athens: and according to many wrote his Chaldæan history in the Greek language. As a priest of Belus he possessed every advantage, which the records of the temple and the learning and traditions of the Chaldæans could afford; and seems to have composed his work with a serious regard for truth. He has sketched his history of the earlier times from the representations on the walls of the temples: from written records and traditionary knowledge, he learned several points too well authenticated to be called in question; and correcting the one by the other has produced the strange history before us.

The first fragment, a catalogue of the Chaldæan Kings, has been preserved by Apollodorus; and the second, another version of the same with an epitome of the account of the deluge, by Abydenus, a disciple of Aristotle. The large extract preserved by Alexander Polyhistor, is extremely valuable; and contains a store of very curious information.

The first book of the history opens naturally enough with a description of Babylonia. Then referring to the paintings, the author finds the first series a kind of preface to the rest. All men of every nation appear assembled in Chaldæa: among them is introduced a character, who is represented as their instructor in the arts and sciences, and informing them of the events, which had previously taken place. Unconscious that Noah is represented under the character of Oannes, Berossus describes him, from the hieroglyphical delineation, as a being literally compounded of a fish and man, and as passing the natural, instead of the diluvian, night in the sea, with other circumstances indicative of his character and life.

The instructions of the Patriarch are detailed in the next series of paintings. In the first of which, I conceive, the Chaos is portrayed by the confusion of the limbs of every kind of animal: the second represents the creation of the universe: the third the formation of mankind: others again that of animals, and of the heavenly bodies.

The second book appears to have comprehended the history of the ante-diluvian world: and in this the two first fragments ought to have been inserted. The historian seems to have confounded the history of the world with that of Chaldæa. He finds nine persons, probably represented as kings, preceding Noah, who is here again introduced under the name of Xisuthrus, and supposes that the representation was of the first dynasty of the Chaldæan kings. From the universal consent of history and tradition he was well assured that Alorus or Orion, the Nimrod of the Scriptures, was the founder of Babylon and the first king: consequently he places him at the top, and Xisuthrus follows as the tenth. The destruction of the records by Nabonasar left him to fill up the intermediate names as he could: and who are inserted, is not so easy to determine. If they are the predecessors of Noah; who are the Annedoti that appear to them? or can these appearances relate to any ante-diluvian transactions of the Patriarch? If they are the successors of Nimrod, the appearances of the Annedoti may refer to visits of the Patriarch and his sons: yet every remnant of the heathen accounts, which in anywise relates to this subject, affirms the violent destruction of the tower of Babel, the dispersion of its builders, and the long subsequent desolation of the city.

There is, however, a dynasty of Chaldæan kings, handed down as some suppose by Berossus, of which the following is a list of the names.

| | | |
|---|---|---|
| 1. Ευηχοος | Evechous | 6 Years. |
| 2. Χομασβολος | Chomasbolus | 7 Years. |
| 3. Πωρος | Porus | 35 Years. |
| 4. Νεχωβης | Nechobes | 43 Years. |
| 5. Αβιος | Abius | 45 Years. |
| 6. Ονιβαλλος | Oniballus | 40 Years. |
| 7. Ζινζιρος | Zinzirus | 45 Years. |

These Mr. Faber conjectures to have been the immediate descendants and successors of Nimrod in Nineveh, the new seat of his empire after the catastrophe at Babylon; and that the long continuation of Assyrian monarchs are the descendants of the same patriarch but of a younger branch. Bryant fancies he recognizes among them the predecessors of Nimrod, and thinks the list altogether spurious.

There is also a dynasty of Arabian kings of Chaldæa, who seem to have taken possession of Babylon during the long period of its desolation, and to have reigned there independent of the Assyrian empire. They were six in number, five of whose names are preserved.

| | | |
|---|---|---|
| 1. Μαρδοκεντης | Mardocentes | 45 Years. |
| 2. Σισιμαδακος | Sisimadacus | 28 Years. |
| 3. Γαβιος | Gabius | 37 Years. |
| 4. Παραννος | Parannus | 40 Years. |
| 5. Ναβοναβος | Nabonnabus | 25 Years. |
| 6. . . . . . . . . . . . . . . | | 41 Years. |

They are to be found in Syncellus.

The history of the flood is very interesting, and wonderfully consonant with the Mosaic account. It mentions also the circuitous route of the human race from Armenia to the plains of Shinar.

The fragment on the Tower of Babel is generally quoted as from Abydenus. Whether it is part of his own work, the Assyrian history, or was extracted by him from Berossus, or transcribed from the Scriptures is extremely questionable: indeed it has much the air of a forgery.

The small fragment (page 32) is supposed by Eusebius, who quotes it, to relate to Abraham. Nor is this improbable: a similar passage is found in Nicolaus Damascenus, which mentions the patriarch by name, and styles him King of Damascus, a title which is given him by other writers.

The other fragments of Berossus are well authenticated history, and throw some light upon the scriptural account of the same persons and transactions. It may be observed that Belshazzar, represented in Daniel, as the son of Nebuchadnezzar, is Neriglissoor, who married the daughter, and afterwards conspired against and slew the son of that monarch; succeeded to the kingdom; and was himself taken off by violence. Nabonnedus corresponds with Darius the Mede, who afterwards took the kingdom, and was conquered by Cyrus.

The last fragment is from Megasthenes, a Persian, who wrote an Indian history a few years subsequently to Berossus. The prophecy of Nebuchadnezzar apparently alludes to some public notification of Daniel's interpretation of his dream. The Mede he mentions may be Nabonnedus, the Darius of the Scripture.

The singular creed, which stands first of the Egyptian fragments, was transcribed by Jamblichus, from the Hermetic books. It is an exposition of that first principle of the heathen theology, which, with its hypostases, was so largely, insisted upon by the school of Plato; and, according to them, so continually passed over in silent reverence by the earliest heathens.

I have retained the translation of Jones of Nayland, from his Philosophical Disquisitions; and which may be found also in his answer to the Essay on Spirit: and I may refer to those works for the most intelligible and satisfactory exposition of this, and of the other heathen trinities.

Previously to the dispersion at Babel, the apostates from the primitive worship were divided into two sects, whose religion Mr. Faber commonly distinguishes by the titles of Buddhism and Brahmenism. They differed not so much in the original objects of their adoration, as in their form of worship. While the latter descended to the introduction of images, and diverged with every kind of polytheistical absurdity; the former stopped content with a more simple scheme of theology; and in some countries, such as Persia, an almost pure Sabianism was jealously preserved. Both were widely diffused and often, as in Egypt and Greece, amalgamated into one. The more elaborate and corrupted system of Brahmenism would catch the attention of the casual observer as the religion of the land; while the deeper doctrines, which involved much of the Buddhic theology, were wrapped in mystery, and communicated only to the initiated.

That the heathen trinities are often variations of the Patriarchs, the Divi of the ancient worship, who were canonized under the titles of Ouranus, Cronus, Jupiter, &c. combined with the ark and other symbols, is demonstrated by Mr. Faber and others, too clearly to admit of doubt: yet, still more frequently, when stripped of their theological dress, will they resolve themselves into some mere physical principle of nature, or its powers: of which the present collection affords other decisive instances both in Sanchoniatho and Zoroaster. Among the ancient heathens the Chaos was an object of veneration; it was looked upon as the first great principle, and usually occupies the first place, in those creeds which bear a trinitarian aspect. The other persons of the Triad are equally material: the second is frequently the Sun, or the Light, or rather Ether, the Soul of the World, or the great Patriarch himself: and the third, the Host of Heaven, the Stars, the Soul of the World, or the consecrated Dæmons. There was a foundation of Materialism, on which was raised a superstructure of Idolatry.

In the classic ages of Greece and Rome appeared a race of philosophers, who, while they submitted to superstitions which they sometimes scorned, must be allowed to have lifted up their minds to truth, as high as unassisted reason might avail. A Christian may despise, as rank idolatry, the weakness or hypocrisy, which could bow down before the images, and pray to the departed spirits of their patriarchal Divi, either as agents or intercessors; but he must admit that their aspirations towards the first great cause soared far above materialism, and were wholly directed to a sublimer object of veneration. By them the ancient creeds were made to speak a loftier language, which was foreign to their original import; and upon the promulgation of Christianity they were again remodelled and refined into a further resemblance of its mysteries. And such has probably been the fate of the Hermetic creed before us.

The old Egyptian Chronicle, preserved by Syncellus, is a valuable guide and index to the dynasties that follow.

The first fragment of Manetho, his Epistle to Ptolemy Philadelphus, king of Egypt, gives an account of the author and his work. His history was composed by order of that king in emulation of the Septuagint: and its materials collected, under the royal command, from all the records of the kingdom. All that remains is an epitome of the dynasties, and two large extracts; the first concerning the Shepherd kings, and the other upon the Israelites.

In the dynasties I have followed the text of Africanus, as quoted by Syncellus, in preference to that of Eusebius who has sadly defaced it. The general outline is the same, though the names of the kings, and the length of their respective reigns frequently differ, as well as the collocation and numbers of the dynasties. I have availed myself of the text of Eusebius to correct grammatical errors; but where any material difference occurs, I have inserted the variation in a parenthesis, or observed it in a note. The numerical letters or figures I have given from Africanus without noticing those of Eusebius as very little dependence can be placed on either.

The Laterculus or Canon of the Kings of Thebes was compiled from the archives of that city by Eratosthenes, the librarian to Ptolemy Philadelphus. It is to be found in Syncellus and other writers.

From these fragments, as explained by the ingenious dissertations of Bryant and Mr. Faber, we may collect an outline of the early history of Egypt. It appears then that after the dispersion from Babel the children of Mizraim went off to Egypt; of which they continued in the undisturbed enjoyment for about two centuries and a half. The first fourteen dynasties have given rise to various hypotheses. Bryant, using the Old Chronicle as an authority, lops them all off at once as spurious. There is nevertheless great reason to suppose that the first, or at least part of it, is genuine. Menes, Mines, or Mizor, the Mizraïm of the Scriptures, and the planter of the nation, is naturally placed as the first sovereign of the united realm: and perhaps the dominion of Athothis was equally extensive; for his name occurs both in the Laterculus of the Theban Kings, and in Sanchoniatho. After him the country seems to have been divided into several independent monarchies; some of whose princes may perhaps be found among the thirteen dynasties that follow.

The first fragment from Josephus, gives an account of the invasion and expulsion of a race of foreigners, who were styled Hycsos or Shepherd Kings. They were a branch of the warlike family of the Cuthites, who took advantage of the divided state of Egypt, and conquered it with little difficulty. They retained possession for nearly two hundred and sixty years; when they were expelled by a combination of the native princes under Thummosis, king of Thebes. The Shepherds are placed as the fifteenth dynasty, and Thummosis and his successors, correspond accurately with Amos the first king and his successors of the eighteenth dynasty. Very shortly after the expulsion of the shepherds, Joseph and the children of Israel, came down into Egypt, and were settled in the land of Goshen, the Avaris, which had been evacuated by the Shepherds; where they seem to have lived more than a century on terms of the greatest amity with the Egyptians, till a second invasion of the Shepherds reduced them to a state of slavery. Of this invasion the second extract gives an account, and places it in the reign of Amenophis, whom the historian identifies with Amenophis the third, by making him the predecessor of Sethos his son, whom we find the first of the nineteenth dynasty, and who was named Ramesses, after Rampses the father of Amenophis. According to the fragment, the Shepherds effected the conquest in alliance with the Israelites, with whom they reigned conjointly thirteen years, during which time Amenophis, with multitudes of his subjects, retired into Ethiopia. By a comparison of the fragment with the Mosaic account, and some passages relative to the same transactions in Diodorus, Herodotus, and Tacitus, Mr. Faber has extracted the following particulars; that instead of thirteen years, one hundred and six must be allotted to the duration of the second shepherd dynasty; the five hundred and eleven years mentioned by Manetho, being the complete interval between the first invasion and final expulsion: that the native Egyptians and Israelites were equally oppressed under their sway: that the Pyramids were constructed by the joint labours of the conquered, at the command of Cheops, one of the Shepherd kings: and that the Exodus of the Israelites, and destruction of the

Shepherd's power were effected at the same time, by the passage of the Red Sea. After the power of the Shepherds was broken by that catastrophe, the native princes returned, and seem to have had some difficulty in expelling the remnant of the Shepherd tribe; which was finally effected by Sethosis, in the emigration of the Danaï to Greece.

The second invasion then must have taken place in the reign of Amenophis the second; and the return of the Egyptian kings from Ethiopia, in the person of Amenophis the third, who has been confounded with his predecessor. The kings of the second dynasty of Shepherds, seem to have been but two, Cheops and Chephren according to Herodotus, the Chemmis and Cephren of Diodorus. They correspond apparently with Suphis, and Suphis the second which are placed in the fourth of the dynasties of Manetho. The second dynasty of Shepherds, was in reality the fourth dynasty of Egypt, which is expressly stated to have been Memphites of a different race: and of these Suphis the first is said by Africanus, to be the same as Cheops. By turning also to the Laterculus we may observe, at the fifteenth, a change of dynasty from Theban Egyptian to Theban kings: and in Saophis and Sensaophis or rather Saophis the second, we may recognise the same persons reigning as the kings of Thebes. The Mencheres of Manetho, who follows Suphis, is probably the Mycerinus of Diodorus and Herodotus, and the Moscheris of Eratosthenes; and a similarity in the names of his successors to those of the successors of Acherres* in the eighteenth, may induce us to suppose they were the same persons, the exiled princes of Egypt, the contemporaries and not the successors of the second race of Shepherd kings. If any reliance may be placed upon the numbers, another argument might be drawn from the sum of the united reigns which amounts in all the three cases to something more than a century. For a very ingenious theory, I may also refer to the Egyptian Mythology of Pritchard, in which he separates the Theban, Memphite, Thinite, Elephantine, Xoïte, and Heracleotic dynasties from each other, and looks upon them as independent and often contemporaneous dynasties.

The Tyrian Annals are fragments, which were quoted by Josephus from the now extinct histories of Dius and Menander. They agree perfectly with the scriptural accounts, and furnish some curious particulars in addition. The date of the foundation of Carthage, it may be observed is accurately fixed.

The fragments of Zoroaster are generally known

* Possibly the name was Cheres or Ares, varied by the common prefixes of Men, Ach, &c.

by the title of the Chaldaic Oracle of Zoroaster. A few of them were first published by Ludovicus Tiletanus at Paris, with the commentaries of Pletho; to which were subsequently added those of Psellus. The rest were collected by Franciscus Patricius from the works of Proclus, Hermias, Simplicius, Damascius, Synesius, Olympiodorus, Nicephorus, and Arnobius; and published together with the Hermetic Books at the end of his Nova Philosophia. Stanley in his lives of the Philosophers, has given the complete collection of the oracles, with a translation into English, to which I have generally adhered.

Great doubts have been entertained respecting the authenticity of these oracles: but the variety of authors by whom they have been quoted, and throughout whose works they lie dispersed, speaks something in their favour. That they were the forgery of some Gnostic, is an opinion which Stanley thinks sufficiently refuted by the great veneration in which they were held by the Platonic school.

The oracles of Zoroaster, if not genuine extracts, at least contain the genuine doctrine of the Sabæan Theology. The writings which are extant under the title of the Hermetic books though of a far more suspicious character, and evidently the compositions of a later age, have by several eminent writers been also supposed to contain the real doctrines of the Egyptian Buddhists. Both savour perhaps too strongly of the Platonic philosophy: but that peculiar phraseology, by which the materiality of their subject is sublimated into a spiritual form, must be attributed to the Greek translators, who had deeply imbibed the doctrines of that school.

The Periplus of Hanno is an account of the earliest voyage of discovery extant. It was taken from an original and apparently official document which was suspended in the temple of Saturn, at Carthage. Mr. Falconer has edited it as a separate work, and gives two dissertations on it; the first, explanatory of its contents; and the second, a refutation of Mr. Dodwell's reflections on its authenticity. I have followed Mr. Falconer both in his text and translation. With respect to its age, Mr. Falconer agrees with Bougainville in referring it to the sixth century before the Christian era.

The Periplus is prefaced by a few lines, reciting a decree of the Carthaginians relative to the voyage and its objects: and is then continued as a narrative, by the commander or one of his companions, which commences from the time the fleet had cleared the straits of Gibraltar. Mr. Bougainville has given a chart of the voyage, which may be found, together with the corresponding maps of Ptolemy and D'Anville, in Mr. Falconer's treatise. It may be sufficient however, to remark that Thymiaterium, the first of the colonies planted by Hanno, occupies a position very nearly, perhaps precisely the same with that of the present commercial city of Mogadore. The promontory of Soloeis corresponds with Cape Bojador, nearly opposite to the Canaries. Caricontichos, Gytte, Acra, Melitta and Arambys are placed between Cape Bojador and the Rio d'Ouro which is supposed to be the Lixus. Cerne is laid down as the island of Arguin under the southern Cape Blanco: the river Chretes perhaps is the St. John, and the next large river mentioned is the Senegal. Cape Palmas and Cape Three Points, are supposed to correspond respectively with the Western and Southern Horns, and some island in the Bight of Benin, with that of the Gorillæ. Vossius however supposes the Western Horn, to be Cape Verd, and the Southern, Cape Palmas, in which case the Sierra Leone will answer to the Ochema Theon the Chariot of the Gods.

The description of the Troglodytæ, as men of a different form or appearance, may imply a change from the Moresco to the Negro race. Some passages, quoted by Mr. Falconer from Bruce's travels, explain the extraordinary fires and nightly merriment, which alarmed the voyagers, as customs common among many of the negro tribes, and which had repeatedly fallen within the scope of his own observations. The Gorillæ are supposed to be large monkeys or wild men as the name ανθρωποι αγριοι may in fact import.

It is needless to take notice of the numerous

forgeries, which have been issued as the productions of the authors of these fragments. There is a complete set which was composed in Latin by Annius, a monk of Viterbo. But it is a singular circumstance, and one which might be urged with great force against the genuineness of almost the whole collection, that not only the original authors have perished, but those also, through whose means these relics have been handed down. With the exception of these fragments, not only have Sanchoniatho, Berossus, and the rest passed on into oblivion; but the preservers of their names have followed in the same track, and to a more unusual fate. The fragments of Philo, Abydenus, Polyhistor, Dius, and the others, are generally not those of their own works, but extracts from their predecessors.

It is necessary also to advert to the numerous errors which will be found in every sheet. The fragments have been exposed to more than the common risks, and accidents, to which all ancient writings have been subject. They have been either copied from the rude annals of antiquity, or sketched from historical paintings or hieroglyphical records, they have been sometimes translated from the sacred, into the common language of the place, and again translated into Greek; then passed in quotation from hand to hand, and are now scattered over the works of the fathers, and the writers of the Roman empire. It is matter of surprise then, not that they abound in error and uncertainty, but that so much has been preserved. For my own errors and inadvertencies I beg leave humbly to apologise, yet I must confess I have some reason to congratulate myself on finding in the above a cloak, under which a multitude of them may be concealed, and to which a charitable disposition may refer as many as it pleases without even recurring to the " errors of the press."

Several of these fragments are preserved in two or three different authors, each of whom contains a different version of the same, differing not so much in the outline, and in the general flow of words, as in those technicalities and variations of termination which were necessary to adapt them to the author's style, and it has been a source of some little perplexity to determine which of these various readings to prefer.

To Eusebius, Syncellus, and Josephus, we are principally indebted for these relics of antiquity. The authors of them are repeatedly cited in the Stromata of Clemens Alexandrinus, and in the works of Justin, Cedrenus, and the fathers of the lower empire: but unfortunately no extracts have been preserved. Diodorus Siculus has borrowed largely, but has incorporated the substance of his quotations in the body of his own work.

For Josephus I have followed Hudson's edition. The Cologne edition of the Præparatio Evangelica of Eusebius is often considered as the best: but upon close inspection and comparison I have been induced to prefer the text of Stephen. With the exception of a mutilated translation into Latin, Eusebius' Chronicle is lost. Under that title however Scaliger has industriously compiled a very portly folio, which, with some other Chronicles, contains a collection of all the fragments of the Greek text of Eusebius, that could be found. Syncellus has been magnificently edited at Paris under the patronage of Louis the fourteenth. By that father very copious extracts have been preserved. He professes to follow the original documents more closely that his predecessors, and as his Parisian editor makes the same pretences to fidelity, I have very generally taken his text as the groundwork. To correct all the palpable grammatical errors contained in it, would be a difficult undertaking. To effect it in some degree, I have availed myself of the emendations of the margin, and of the different readings to be found in Eusebius. But in no case have I presumed to alter without authority; and where neither the margin nor Eusebius afforded that, I have permitted the error to stand as I found it. The alteration of a single letter would sometimes correct a gross grammatical mistake: yet at the same time by retaining the letters as they stand, and making a different division of them into words, a different meaning may be elicited. This work being a mere collection of quotations,

I have not deviated from the usual method of quoting without the points. In most cases we make no use of them: in some instances, their introduction might stamp one particular signification upon certain passages, in which two, widely different, present themselves: but where so much uncertainty prevails, every person must be at liberty to accent as he pleases, or to divide the words as best may suit his purpose. To introduce the accents generally, and omit them in those sentences which may bear a double import, and in which they might assist us to determine the meaning; in short, to use them where they are of no use, and omit them where they might be turned to some account, would be an eccentricity, more needing an apology, than the course I have ventured to pursue. The matter contained in these fragments is the only merit to which they can pretend; the interpretation is all that is required; and refined criticism, bestowed on works which do not rise to elegance, is always a misplaced display of learning: and I feel myself as little competent as inclined to enter into speculations upon the words or accents. So far from presuming to intrude into the province of a commentator, I shall be well content if I have committed no great mistakes.

Such as these fragments are, I send them forth without either note or comment. The classical reader will find, I fear, but poor amusement in perusing a half barbarous dialect, replete with errors and inconsistencies: to the student of divinity, however, they may not be altogether unacceptable or devoid of interest: and to the inquirer after ancient history and mythology, it may be useful to have collected into one small volume, the scattered relics for which he must otherwise search so widely.

THE

# THEOLOGY OF THE PHŒNICIANS;

FROM

# SANCHONIATHO.

# SANCHONIATHO.

## THE COSMOGONY.

ΤΗΝ των ὁλων αρχην ὑποτιθεται Αερα ζοφωδη και πνευματωδη, η πνοην αερος ζοφωδους, και Χαος θολερον, ερεβωδες· ταυτα δε ειναι απειρα, και δια πολυν αιωνα μη εχειν περας. ὁτε δε (φησιν) ηρασθη το πνευμα των ιδιων αρχων, και εγενετο συγκρασις, ἡ πλοκη εκεινη εκληθη Ποθος. αὑτη δε αρχη κτισεως ἁπαντων. αυτο δε ουκ εγινωσκε την αυτου κτισιν, και εκ της αυτου συμπλοκης του πνευματος, εγενετο Μωτ. τουτο τινες φασιν ιλυν. οἱ δε, ὑδατωδους μιξεως σηψιν. και εκ ταυτης εγενετο πασα σπορα κτισεως, και γενεσις των ὁλων.

Ην δε τινα ζωα ουκ εχοντα αισθησιν, εξ ὡν εγενετο ζωα

He supposes that the beginning of all things was a dark and condensed windy air, or a breeze of dark air and a Chaos turbid and indistinct like Erebus: and that these things were infinite, and for a long time had no bound: but when this wind became enamoured of its own principles, and a mixture took place, that embrace was called Desire: and it was the beginning of the creation of all things. But the wind knew not its own production. And of that wind from its embrace was begotten Môt; which some call Mud, others the putrefaction of a watery mixture: and from this sprung all the seed of the creation, and the generation of the universe.

But there were certain animals which had no sense, out of which proνοερα, και εκληθη Ζωφασημιν, τουτ' εστιν ουρανου κατοπται. και ανεπλασθη ὁμοιως ὠου σχηματι, και εξελαμψε Μωτ, Ἡλιος τε και Σεληνη, Αστερες τε και Αστρα μεγαλα.

ceeded intelligent animals, and they were called Zophasemin, that is, the inspectors of heaven, and they were moulded in like manner in the shape of an egg, and Môt shone forth the sun and the moon, the less and the greater stars.

Και του αερος διαυγαζαντος, δια πυρωσιν και της θαλασσης και της γης εγενετο πνευματα, και νεφη, και ουρανιων ὑδατων μεγισται καταφοραι και χυσεις και επειδη διεκριθη, και του ιδιου τοπου διεχωρισθη δια την του ἡλιου πυρωσιν, και παντα συνηντησε παλιν εν αερι ταδε τοισδε, και συνεῤῥαξαν, βρονται τε απετελεσθησαν και αστραπαι, και προς τον παταγον των βροντων τα προγεγραμμενα νοερα ζωα εγρηγορησεν, και προς τον ηχον επτυρη, και εκινηθη εν τη γη και θαλασση αῤῥεν και θηλυ.

And the air shining thoroughly with light, by its fiery influence on the sea and earth, winds were produced, and clouds, and very great defluxions, and torrents of the heavenly waters. And when these things, by the heat of the sun, were parted and separated from their proper places, and all met again in the air, and were dashed to pieces against each other, thunders and lightnings were the effect; and at the sound of the thunders, the before-mentioned intelligent animals were awakened, and frightened by the noise, and male and female moved upon the earth, and in the sea.

(Τουτοις ἑξης ὁ αυτος συγγραφευς επιφερει λεγων.) ταυθ' εὑρεθη εν τη κοσμογονια γεγραμμενα Taαυτου, και τοις εκεινου ὑπομνημασιν, εκ τε στοχασμων και τεκμηριων, ὡν ἑωρακεν αυτου ἡ διανοια, και εὑρε, και ἡμιν εφωτισεν.

(After these things our Author proceeds to say:) These things are written in the Cosmogony of Taautus, and in his n emoirs, and from the conjectures, and natural signs which his mind perceived and discovered, and wherewith he has enlightened us.

Ἑξης τουτοις ονοματα των ανεμων ειπων Νοτου και Βορεου και των λοιπων, επιλεγει.

Afterwards, declaring the names of the winds North, South, and the rest, he makes this epilogue:—But these

Αλλ' οὑτοιγε πρωτοι αφιερωσαντα τα της γης βλαστηματα, και θεους ενομισαν, και προσεκυνουν ταυτα, αφ' ὡν αυτοι τε διεγινοντο, και οἱ επομενοι, και οἱ προ αυτων παντες, και χοας και επιθυσεις εποιουν. (και επιλεγει) αἱται δε ησαν αἱ επινοιαι της προσκυνησεως, ὁμοιαι τῃ αυτων ασθενειᾳ και ψυχης ατολμιᾳ.

first men consecrated the plants of the earth, and judged them gods, and worshipped those things, upon which they themselves lived, and all their posterity, and all before them; to these they made libations and sacrifices. Then he proceeds:—Such were the devices of worship, agreeing with their weakness and the want of boldness of their souls.—*Euseb. Præp. Evan.* lib. I. c. 10.

## THE GENERATIONS.

Ειτα (φησι) γεγενησθαι εκ του Κολπια ανεμου, και γυναικος αυτου Βααυ, τουτο δε νυκτα ἑρμηνευειν, Αιωνα και Πρωτογονον θνητους ανδρας, οὑτω καλουμενους, εὑρειν δε τον Αιωνα την απο των δενδρων τροφην.

Of the wind Colpias, and his wife Baau, which is interpreted Night, were begotten two mortals, called Æon and Protogonus: and Æon found out food from trees.

Εκ τουτων τους γενομενους κληθηναι Γενος και Γενεαν, και οικησαι την Φοινικην. αυχμων δε γενομενων, τας χειρας ορεγειν εις ουρανους προς τον Ἡλιον. τουτον γαρ (φησι) θεον ενομιζον μονον ουρανου Κυριον, Βεελσαμην καλουντες, ὁ εστι παρα Φοινιξι κυριος ουρανου, Ζευς δε παρ' Ἑλλησι.

Those that were begotten of these were called Genus and Genea, and they dwelt in Phœnicia: and when there were great droughts they stretched forth their hands to heaven towards the Sun: for him they thought the only lord of heaven, calling him Beelsamin, which in Phœnician is Lord of Heaven, but in the Greek Zeus.

Ἑξης (φησιν) απο Γενους Αιωνος και Πρωτογονου, γενη-

Afterwards by Genus, the son of Protogonus and Æon, were begotten θηναι αυθις παιδας θνητας, οἱς ειναι ονοματα Φως και Πυρ και Φλοξ. οὑτοι (φησιν) εκ παρατριψης ξυλων εὑρον πυρ, και την χρησιν εδιδαξαν.

Υἱους δε εγεννησαν οὑτοι μεγεθει τε και ὑπεροχῃ κρεισσονας. ὡν τα ονοματα τοις ορεσιν επετεθη ὡν εκρατησαν. ὡς εξ αυτων κληθηναι το Κασσιον, και τον Λιβανον, και τον Αντιλιβανον, και το Βραθυ.

Εκ τουτων (φησιν) εγεννηθησαν Μημρουμος ὁ και Ὑψουρανιος απο μητερων δε (φησιν,) εχρηματιζοντων τοτε γυναικων αναιδην μισγομενων οἱς αν εντυχοιεν. Ειτα (φησι) τον Ὑψουρανιον οικησαι Τυρον, καλυβας τε επινοησαι απο καλαμων και θρυων, και παπυρων. στασιασαι δε προς τον αδελφον Ουσωον. ὁς σκεπην τῳ σωματι πρωτος εκ δερματων, ὡν ισχυσε συλλαβειν θηριων εὑρε. Ῥαγδαιων δε γενομενων ομβρων και πνευματων, παρατριβεντα τα εν τῃ Τυρῳ δενδρα, πυρ αναψαι, και την αυτοθι ὑλην καταφλεξαι. δενδρου δε λαβομενον τον Ουσωον και αποκλαδευσαντα, πρωτον τολμησαι εις θαλασσαν εμβηναι· ανιερωσαι δε δυο στηλας πυρι τε και πνευματι, και προσκυνησαι, ἁμα τε σπενδειν

mortal children, whose names were Phôs, Púr, and Phlox. These found out the method of producing fire by rubbing pieces of wood against each other, and taught men the use thereof.

These begat sons of vast bulk and height, whose names were given to the mountains on which they first seised: thus from them were named Mount Cassius, and Libanus, Antilibanus, and Brathu.

Memrumus and Hypsuranius were the issue of these men having intercourse with their mothers, the women of those times, without shame, lying with any man they chanced to meet. Then Hypsuranius inhabited Tyre: and he invented the making of huts of reeds and rushes, and the papyrus. And he fell into enmity with his brother Usous, who first made clothing for the body of the skins of the wild beasts which he could catch. And when there were violent storms of rain and wind, the trees in Tyre being rubbed against each other, took fire, and the forest there was consumed. And Usous having taken a tree, and broken off its boughs, first dared to venture on the sea. And he consecrated two pillars to Fire and Wind, and worshipped them, and poured out to them the blood of the wild beasts he took in hunting: and when there was an end of these (the storm and fire?)

αυταις εξ ὧν ἤγρευε θηριων. τουτων δε τελευτησαντων, τους απολειφθεντας (φησι) ῥαβδους αυτοις αφιερωσαι, και τας στηλας προσκυνειν, και τουτοις ἑορτας αγειν κατ᾽ ετος.

he consecrated to them the stumps of wood that remained, and worshipped the pillars, and held anniversary feasts unto the stumps.

Χρονοις δε ὑστερον πολλοις απο της Ὑψουρανιου γενεας γενεσθαι Αγρεα και Ἁλιεα, τους ἁλειας και αγρας εὑρετας. εξ ὧν κληθηναι αγρευτας και ἁλιεις.

And in the times after the generation of Hypsuranius, were Agreus and Halieus, the inventors of the arts of hunting and fishing, from whom huntsmen and fishermen are named.

Εξ ὧν γενεσθαι δυο αδελφους σιδηρου εὑρετας, και της τουτου εργασιας. ὧν θατερον τον Χρυσωρ λογους ασκησαι, και επῳδας και μαντειας. ειναι δε τουτον τον Ἡφαιστον. εὑρειν δε και αγκιστρον, και δελεαρ, και ὁρμιαν, και σχεδιαν· πρωτον τε παντων ανθρωπων πλευσαι. διο και ὡς Θεον αυτον μετα θανατον εσεβασθησαν. καλεισθαι δε αυτον και Διαμιχιον. οἱ δε τους αδελφους αυτου τοιχους φασιν επινοησαι εκ πλινθων.

Of these were begotten two brothers who discovered iron, and the forging thereof. One of these called Chrysor, who is the same with Hephæstus, exercised himself in words, and charms, and divinations; and he invented the hook, bait, and fishing-line, and boats slightly built; and he was the first of all men that sailed. Wherefore he was worshipped after his death as a God, and called Diamichius. And it is said his brothers invented the way of making walls of bricks.

Μετα ταυτ᾽ εκ του γενους τουτου γενεσθαι νεανιδας δυο, καλεισθαι δε αυτων τον μεν Τεχνιτην· τον δε Γηϊνον Αυτοχθονα. οὗτοι επενοησαν τῳ πηλῳ της πλινθου συμμιγνυειν φορυτον, και τῳ ἡλιῳ αυτας τερσαινειν. αλλα και στεγας εξευρον.

Afterwards, from this generation were born two youths, one of whom was called Technites, the other Geïnus Autochthôn. These discovered the method of mingling stubble with the loam of the bricks, and of drying them in the sun; and found out tiling.

Απο τουτων εγενοντο ἑτεροι, ὡν ὁ μεν Αγρος εκαλειτο. ὁ δε Αγρουηρος η Αγροτης. οὑ και ξοανον ειναι μαλα σεβασμιον, και ναον ζυγοφορουμενον εν Φοινικη. παρα δε Βιβλιοις εξαιρετως θεων ὁ μεγιστος ονομαζεται. επινοησαν δε οὑτοι αυλας προστιθεναι τοις οικοις, και περιβολαια, και σπηλαια. εκ τουτων αγροται και κυνηγοι. οὑτοι δε και Αληται και Τιτανες καλουνται.

By these were begotten others, of which one was called Agrus, the other Agrouerus or Agrotes, of whom in Phœnicia there was a statue held in the highest veneration, and a temple drawn by yokes of oxen: and at Byblus he is called, by way of eminence, the greatest of the Gods. These invented courts, and fences for houses, and caves or cellars: husbandmen, and such as hunt with dogs, derive their origin from these: they are called also Aletæ, and Titans.

Απο τουτων γενεσθαι Αμυνον και Μαγον. οἱ κατεδειξαν κωμας και ποιμνας.

From these were descended Amynus and Magus, who taught men to construct villages and tend flocks.

Απο τουτων γενεσθαι Μισωρ και Συδυκ. τουτ᾽ εστιν ευλυτον και δικαιον. οὑτοι την του ἁλος χρησιν εὑρον.

By these men were begotten Misor and Sydyc, that is, Well-freed and Just: and they found out the use of salt.

Απο Μισωρ Τααυτος. ὁς εὑρε την των πρωτων στοιχειων γραφην. ὁν Αιγυπτιοι μεν Θωωρ, Αλεξανδρεις δε Θωυθ, Ἑλληνες δ᾽ Ἑρμην εκαλεσαν. εκ δε του Συδυκ, Διοσκουροι, η Καβειροι, η Κορυβαντες. η Σαμοθρακες. οὑτοι (φησι) πρωτοι πλοιον εὑρον.

From Misor came Taautus, who invented the writing of the first letters; him the Egyptians called Thoor, the Alexandrians Thoyth, and the Greeks Hermes. But from Sydyc came the Dioscuri, or Cabiri, or Corybantes, or Samothraces: these (he says) first built a ship complete.

Εκ τουτων γεγονασιν ἑτεροι, οἱ και βοτανας εὑρον, και την των δακετων ιασιν, και επῳδας.

From these descended others, who discovered medicinal herbs, and the cure of poisons and charms.

Κατα τουτους γινεται τις Ελιουν καλουμενος Ὑψιστος· και θηλεια λεγομενη Βηρουθ.

Contemporary with these was one Elioun, which imports Hypsistus, (the most high) and his wife called οἱ και κατῳκουν περι Βυβλον. εξ ὡν γενεται Επιγειος η Αυτοχθων. ὁν ὑστερον εκαλεσαν Ουρανον. ὡς απ' αυτου και το ὑπερ ἡμας στοιχειον, δι' ὑπερβολην του καλλους ονομαζειν Ουρανον. γενεται δε τουτῳ αδελφη εκ των προειρημενων. ἡ δε εκληθη Γη. και δια το καλλος, απ' αυτης (φησιν) εκαλεσαν την ὁμωνυμον Γην.

Berath, and they dwelt about Byblus; of whom was begotten Epigeus or Autochthon, whom they afterwards called Ouranus (Heaven); so that from him that element, which is over us, by reason of its excellent beauty is named heaven: and he had a sister of the same parents, and she was called Ge (Earth), and by reason of her beauty the earth was called by the same name.

Ὁ δε τουτων πατηρ ὁ Ὑψιστος εκ συμβολης θηριων τελευτησας αφιερωθη. ᾡ και χοας και θυσιας οἱ παιδες ετελεσαν.

Hypsistus, the father of these, having been killed in a conflict with wild beasts, was consecrated, and his children offered libations and sacrifices unto him.

Παραλαβων δε ὁ Ουρανος την του πατρος αρχην, αγεται προς γαμον την αδελφην Γην, και ποιειται εξ αυτης παιδας δ'. Ιλον, τον και Κρονον, και Βετυλον, και Δαγων, ὁς εστι σιτων, και Ατλαντα.

But Ouranus, taking the kingdom of his father, married his sister Ge, and had by her four sons, Ilus who is called Cronus, and Betylus, and Dagon who is Siton, and Atlas.

Και εξ αλλων δε γαμετων ὁ Ουρανος πολλην εσχε γενεαν. διο και χαλεπαινουσα ἡ Γη, τον Ουρανον ζηλοτυπουσα εκακιζεν, ὡς και διαστηναι αλληλων. ὁ δε Ουρανος αποχωρησας αυτης μετα βιας, ὁτε και εβουλετο επιων' και πλησιαζων αυτῃ, παλιν απηλλατετο. επεχειρει δε και τους εξ αυτης παιδας διαφθειρειν. την δε Γην αμυνασθαι πολλακις, συμμαχιαν αυτῃ συλλεξαμενην.

But by other wives Ouranus had much issue; whereat Ge, being grieved and jealous, reproached Ouranus, so that they parted from each other: but Ouranus, though he had parted from her, yet by force returned whenever he pleased, and having laid with her again departed; moreover he attempted to kill the children he had by her; Ge also often defended or avenged herself, gathering unto her auxiliary powers.

Εις ανδρας δε προελθων ὁ Κρονος Ἑρμῃ τῳ τρισμεγιστῳ συμβουλῳ και βοηθῳ χρωμενος, οὗτος γαρ ην αυτου γραμματευς, τον πατερα Ουρανον αμυνεται, τιμωρων τῃ μητρι. Κρονου δε γινονται παιδες, Περσεφονη και Αθηνα. ἡ μεν ουν πρωτη, παρθενος ετελευτα. της δε Αθηνας γνωμῃ και Ἑρμου κατεσκευασε Κρονος εκ σιδηρου ἁρπην και δορυ. Ειτα ὁ Ἑρμης τοις του Κρονου συμμαχοις λογους μαγειας διαλεχθεις, ποθον ενεποιησε τοις κατ' Ουρανου μαχης ὑπερ της Γης. και οὑτω Κρονος τον Ουρανον πολεμῳ συμβαλων, της αρχης ηλασε, και την βασιλειαν διεδεξατο. Ἑαλω δε εν τῃ μαχῃ και ἡ επεραστος του Ουρανου συγκοιτος εγκυμων ουσα· ἡν εκδιδωσιν ὁ Κρονος προς γαμον τῳ Δαγωνι. τικτει δε παρα τουτῳ ὁ κατα γαστρος εξ Ουρανου εφερεν· ὁ δε εκαλεσε Δημαρουν.

But when Cronus came to man's age, by the advice and assistance of Hermes Trismegistus, who was his secretary, he opposed his father Ouranus, that he might avenge his mother. And Cronus had children, Persephone and Athena; the former died a virgin; but, by the advice of Athena and Hermes, Cronus made of iron a scimitar and a spear. Then Hermes, addressing the allies of Cronus with magic words, wrought in them a keen desire to fight against Ouranus in behalf of Ge. And thus Cronus overcoming Ouranus in battle, drove him from his kingdom, and succeeded him in the imperial power. In the battle was taken a well-beloved concubine of Ouranus who was pregnant; Cronus gave her in marriage to Dagon, and she was delivered, and called the child Demaroon.

Επι τουτοις ὁ Κρονος τειχος περιβαλλει τῃ ἑαυτου οικησει, και πρωτην πολιν κτιζει την επι Φοινικης Βυβλον. Μετα ταυτα τον αδελφον τον ιδιον Ατλαντα ὑπονοησας ὁ Κρονος, μετα γνωμης του Ἑρμου εις βαθος γης εμβαλων κατεχωσε.

After these events Cronus builds a wall round about his habitation, and founds Byblus, the first city of Phoenicia. Afterwards Cronus suspecting his own brother Atlas, by the advice of Hermes, threw him into a deep cavern in the earth, and buried him.

Κατα τουτον τον χρονον οἱ

At this time the descendants of the

απο των Διοσκουρων σχεδιας και πλοια συνθεντες, επλευσαν. και εκριφεντες κατα το Κασσιον ορος, ναον αυτοθι αφιερωσαν.

Dioscuri, having built some light and other more complete ships, put to sea; and being cast out over against Mount Cassius, there consecrated a temple.

Οἱ δε συμμαχοι Ἰλου του Κρονου Ελωειμ επεκληθησαν, ὡς αν Κρονιοι· ουτοι ησαν οἱ λεγομενοι επι Κρονου. Κρονος δε υἱον εχων Σαδιδον, ιδιῳ αυτον σιδηρῳ διεχρησατο, δι' ὑπονοιας αυτον εσχηκως· και της ψυχης, αυτοχειρ του παιδος γενομενος, εστερησεν. ὡσαυτως και θυγατρος ιδιας την κεφαλην απετεμεν· ὡς παντας εκπεπληχθαι θεους την Κρονου γνωμην.

But the auxiliaries of Ilus, who is Cronus, were called Eloim, (as it were) the allies of Cronus; they were so called after Cronus. And Cronus, having a son called Sadidus, dispatched him with his own sword, because he held him in suspicion, and with his own hand deprived his son of life. And in like manner he cut off the head of his own daughter, so that all the gods were amazed at the mind of Cronus.

Χρονου δε προϊοντος Ουρανος εν φυγῃ τυγχανων, θυγατερα αυτου παρθενον Ασταρτην μεθ' ἑτερων αυτης αδελφων δυο, Ῥεας και Διωνης, δολῳ τον Κρονον ανελειν ὑποπεμπει· ἁς και ἑλων ὁ Κρονος κουριδιας γαμετας αδελφας ουσας εποιησατο. Γνους δε ὁ Ουρανος, επιστρατευει κατα του Κρονου Ειμαρμενην και Ὡραν μεθ' ἑτερων συμμαχων. και ταυτας εξοικειωσαμενος ὁ Κρονος, παρ' ἑαυτῳ κατεσχεν. ετι δε (φησιν) επενοησε θεος Ουρανος Βαιτυλια, λιθους εμψυχους μηχανησαμενος.

But in process of time, Ouranus being in banishment, sent his daughter Astarte, with two other sisters, Rhea and Dione, to cut off Cronus by deceit; but Cronus took the damsels, and married them being his own sisters. Ouranus, understanding this, sent Eimarmene and Hora with other auxiliaries to make war against him: but Cronus gained the affections of these also, and kept them with himself. Moreover, the god Ouranus devised Bætulia, contriving stones that moved as having life.

Κρονῳ δε εγενοντο απο

And Cronus begat on Astarte seven

Ασταρτης θυγατερες ἑπτα Τιτανιδες η Αρτεμιδες. και παλιν τῳ αυτῳ γινονται απο Ῥεας παιδες ἑπτα, ὧν ὁ νεωτατος ἁμα τη γενεσει αφιερωθη, και απο Διωνης θηλειαι, και απο Ασταρτης παλιν αῤῥενες δυο, Ποθος και Ερως.

daughters called Titanides, or Artemides; and he begat on Rhea seven sons, the youngest of whom was consecrated from his birth; also by Dione he had daughters, and by Astarte moreover two sons, Pothos and Eros.

Ὁ δε Δαγων επειδη εὑρε σιτον και αροτρον, εκληθη Ζευς Αροτριος.

And Dagon, after he had found out bread-corn and the plough, was called Zeus Arotrius.

Συδυκῳ δε τῳ λεγομενῳ δικαιῳ, μια των Τιτανιδων συνελθουσα, γεννα τον Ασκληπιον. εγεννηθησαν δε και εν Περαιᾳ Κρονῳ, τρεις παιδες, Κρονος ὁμωνυμος τῳ πατρι, και Ζευς Βηλος, και Απολλων.

To Sydyc, called the just, one of the Titanides bare Asclepius: Cronus had also in Peræa three sons, Cronus bearing his father's name, and Zeus Belus, and Apollo.

Κατα τουτους γινονται Ποντος και Τυφων και Νηρευς, πατηρ Ποντου. απο δε του Ποντου γινεται Σιδων· ἡ καθ' ὑπερβολην ευφωνιας πρωτη ὑμνον ᾠδης εὑρε. και Ποσειδων.

Contemporary with these were Pontus, and Typhon, and Nereus the father of Pontus: from Pontus descended Sidon, who by the excellence of her singing first invented the hymns of odes or praises: and Posidon.

Τῳ δε Δημαροοντι γινεται Μελικαρθος. ὁ και Ἡρακλης.

But to Demaroon was born Melicarthus, who is also called Heracles.

Ειτα παλιν Ουρανος πολεμει Ποντῳ. και αποστας, Δημαροοντι προστιθεται. Επεισι τε Ποντῳ ὁ Δημαρους, τρεπεται τε αυτον ὁ Ποντος. ὁ δε Δημαρους φυγης θυσιαν ηυξατο.

Then again Ouranus makes war against Pontus, but parting from him attaches himself to Demaroon. Demaroon invades Pontus, but Pontus puts him to flight, and Demaroon vows a sacrifice for his escape.

Ετει δε τριακοστῳ δευτερῳ της ἑαυτου κρατησεως και βασιλειας, ὁ Ιλος, τουτ' εστιν

In the thirty-second year of his power and reign, Ilus, who is Cronus, having laid an ambuscade for his ὁ Κρονος, Ουρανον τον πατερα λοχησας εν τοπῳ τινι μεσογειῳ, και λαβων ὑποχειριον, εκτεμνει αυτου τα αιδοια, συνεγγυς πηγων τε και ποταμων. ενθα αφιερωθη Ουρανος, και απηρτισθη αυτου το πνευμα, και απεσταξεν αυτου το αἱμα των αιδοιων, εις τας πηγας, και των ποταμων τα ὑδατα, και μεχρι τουτου δεικνυται το χωριον.

(Παλιν δε ὁ συγγραφευς τουτοις επιφερει μεθ' ἑτερα λεγων.) Ασταρτη δε ἡ μεγιστη, και Ζευς Δημαρους, και Αδωδις βασιλευς θεων, εβασιλευον της χωρας, Κρονου γνωμη. ἡ δε Ασταρτη επεθηκε τη ιδιᾳ κεφαλῃ βασιλειας παρασημον κεφαλην ταυρου. περινοστουσα δε την οικουμενην, εὑρεν αεροπετη αστερα, ὁν και ανελομενη, εν Τυρῳ τῃ ἁγιᾳ νησῳ αφιερωσε. (Την δε Ασταρτην Φοινικες, την Αφροδιτην ειναι λεγουσι.)

Και ὁ Κρονος δε περιιων την οικουμενην, Αθηνᾳ τῃ ἑαυτου θυγατρι διδωσι της Αττικης την βασιλειαν. λοιμου δε γενομενου και φθορας, τον ἑαυτου μονογενη υἱον, Κρονος Ουρανῳ πατρι ὁλοκαρποι, και τα αιδοια περιτεμνεται, ταυτο ποιησαι και τους ἁμ' αυτῳ συμμαχους

father Ouranus in a certain place in the middle of the earth, and having gotten him into his hands, dismembers him near fountains and rivers. There Ouranus was consecrated, and his spirit was separated, and the blood of his parts dropt into the fountains and the waters of the rivers; and the place is showed even to this day.

(Then our historian, after some other things, goes on thus:) But Astarte called the greatest, and Demaroon entitled Zeus, and Adodus named the king of gods, reigned over the country by the consent of Cronus: and Astarte put upon her head, as the mark of her sovereignty, a bull's head: and travelling about the habitable world, she found a star falling through the air, which she took up, and consecrated in the holy island Tyre: and the Phœnicians say that Astarte is Aphrodite.

Cronus, also going about the habitable world, gave to his daughter Athena the kingdom of Attica: and when there happened a plague and mortality, Cronus offered up his only son as a sacrifice to his father Ouranus, and circumcised himself, and forced his allies to do the same: and not long afterwards he consecrated καταναγκασας. και μετ' ου πολυ έτερον αυτου παιδα απο Ῥέας ονομαζομενον Μουθ' αποθανοντα αφιεροι. Θανατον δε τουτον και Πλουτωνα Φοινικες ονομαζουσι.

Και επι τουτοις ὁ Κρονος Βυβλον μεν την πολιν θεα Βααλτιδι, τη και Διωνη διδωσι. Βηρυτον δε Ποσειδωνι και Καβειροις αγροταις τε και άλιευσιν. οἱ και Ποντου λειψανα, εις την Βηρυτον αφιερωσαν.

Προ δε τουτων θεος Taαυτος μιμησαμενος τον Ουρανον, των θεων οψεις, Κρονου τε και Δαγωνος, και των λοιπων διετυπωσεν τους ἱερους των στοιχειων χαρακτηρας. επενοησε δε και τω Κρονω παρασημα βασιλειας, ομματα τεσσαρα εκ των εμπροσθιων και των οπισθιων μερων· δυο δε ἡσυχη μυοντα· και επι των ωμων πτερα τεσσαρα· δυο μεν, ὡς ἱπταμενα, δυο δε ὡς ὑφειμενα. το δε συμβολον ην, επειδη Κρονος κοιμωμενος εβλεπε, και εγρηγορως εκοιματο· και επι των πτερων ὁμοιως· ότι αναπαυομενος ἱπτατο, και ἱπταμενος ανεπαυετο. τοις δε λοιποις θεοις, δυο ἑκαστω πτερωματα επι των ωμων, ὡς ότι δη συνιπταντο τω Κρονω. και αὐτω δε παλιν επι της κεφαλης,

after his death another son, called Muth, whom he had by Rhea; him the Phœnicians call Death and Pluto.

After these things, Cronus gives the city of Byblus to the goddess Baaltis, which is Dione, and Berytus to Posidon, and to the Caberi, the husbandmen and fishermen: and they consecrated the remains of Pontus at Berytus.

But before these things the god Taautus, having represented Ouranus, made types of the countenances of the gods Cronus, and Dagon, and the sacred characters of the other elements. He contrived also for Cronus the ensign of his royal power, having four eyes in the parts before and in the parts behind, two of them closing as in sleep; and upon the shoulders four wings, two in the act of flying, and two reposing as at rest. And the symbol was, that Cronus whilst he slept was watching, and reposed whilst he was awake. And in like manner with respect to his wings, that whilst he rested he was flying, yet rested whilst he flew. But to the other gods there were two wings only to each upon his shoulders, to intimate that they flew under the controul of Cronus; he had also two wings upon his head, the one for πτερα δυο. ἑν επι του ἡγεμονικωτατου νου, και ἑν επι της αισθησεως.

the most governing part, the mind, and one for the sense.

Ελθων δε ὁ Κρονος εις νοτου χωραν, ἁπασαν την Αιγυπτον εδωκε θεῳ Τααυτῳ, ὁπως βασιλειον αυτῳ γενηται.

And Cronus coming into the country of the south, gave all Egypt to the god Taautus, that it might be his kingdom.

Ταυτα δε (φησι) πρωτοι αυτων ὑπεμνηματισαντο οἱ ἑπτα Συδεκ παιδες Καβηροι, και ογδοος αυτων αδελφος Ασκληπιος, ὡς αυτοις ενετειλατο θεος Τααυτος.

These things, says he, the Caberi, the seven sons of Sydec, and their eighth brother Asclepius, first of all set down in memoirs, as the god Taautus commanded them.

Ταυτα παντα ὁ Θαβιωνος παις, πρωτος των απ' αιωνος γεγονοτων Φοινικων Ἱεροφαντης αλληγορησας, τοις τε φυσικοις και κοσμικοις παθεσιν αναμιξας, παρεδωκε τοις οργιωσι, και τελετων καταρχουσι προφηταις. οἱ τον τυφον αυξειν εκ παντος επινοουντες, τοις αυτων διαδοχοις παρεδωσαν και τοις επεισακτοις. ὡν εἱς ην και Ισιρις των τριων γραμματων εὑρετης, αδελφος Χνα του πρωτου μετονομασθεντος Φοινικος.

All these things the son of Thabion, the first Hierophant of all among the Phœnicians, allegorized and mixed up with the occurrences and passions of nature and the world, and delivered to the priests and prophets, the superintendants of the mysteries: and they, perceiving the rage for these allegories increase, delivered them to their successors, and to foreigners: of whom one was Isiris, the inventor of the three letters, the brother of Chna, who is called the first Phœnician.—*Euseb. Præp. Evan.* lib. I. c. 10.

## OF THE MYSTICAL SACRIFICE OF THE EGYPTIANS.

Εθος ην τοις παλαιοις, εν ταις μεγαλαις συμφοραις των κινδυνων, αντι της παντων φθορας, το ηγαπημενον των τεκνων, τους κρατουντας η

It was the custom among the ancients, in times of great calamity, to prevent the ruin of all, for the rulers of the city or nation to sacrifice to the avenging deities the most beloved πολεως η εθνους, εις σφαγην επιδιδοναι λυτρον τοις τιμωροις δαιμοσι. κατεσφαττοντο δε οἱ διδομενοι μυστικως. Κρονος τοινυν, ὁν οἱ Φοινικες Ισραηλ (Ιλ.?) προσαγορευουσι, βασιλευων της χωρας, και ὑστερον μετα την του βιου τελευτην εις τον του Κρονου αστερα καθιερωθεις, εξ επιχωριας νυμφης Ανωβρετ λεγομενης, υἱον εχων μονογενη, ὁν δια τουτο Ιεουδ εκαλουν, του μονογενους οὑτως ετι και νυν καλουμενου παρα τοις Φοινιξι, κινδυνων εκ πολεμου μεγιστων κατειληφοτων την χωραν, βασιλικῳ κοσμησας σχηματι τον υἱον, βωμον τε κατασκευασαμενος κατεθυσεν.

of their children as the price of redemption: they who were devoted for this purpose were offered mystically. For Cronus, whom the Phœnicians call Il, and who after his death was deified and instated in the planet which bears his name, when king, had by a nymph of the country called Anobret an only son, who on that account is styled Ieoud, for so the Phœnicians still call an only son: and when great danger from war beset the land he adorned the altar, and invested this son with the emblems of royalty, and sacrificed him. —*Euseb. Præp. Evan.* lib. I. c. 10.

## OF THE SERPENT.

Την μεν ουν του δρακοντος φυσιν και των οφεων αυτος εξεθειασεν ὁ Ταautος, και μετ' αυτον αυθις Φοινικες τε και Αιγυπτιοι. πνευματικωτατον γαρ το ζωον παντων των ἑρπετων, και πυρωδες ὑπ' αυτου παρεδοθη. παρ' ᾧ και ταχος ανυπερβλητον δια του πνευματος παριστησι, χωρις ποδων τε και χειρων, η αλλου τινος των εξωθεν, εξ ὡν τα λοιπα ζωα τας κινησεις ποιειται. και

Taautus first consecrated the basilisk, and introduced the worship of the serpent tribe; in which he was followed by the Phœnicians and Egyptians. For this animal was held by him to be the most inspirited of all the reptiles, and of a fiery nature; inasmuch as it exhibits an incredible celerity, moving by its spirit without either hands, or feet, or any of those external organs, by which other animals effect their motion. And in its progress it assumes a variety of forms, moving in a ποικιλων σχηματων τυπους αποτελει, και κατα την πορειαν ἑλικοειδεις εχει τας ὁρμας, εφ' ὁ βουλεται ταχος· και πολυχρονιωτατον δε εστι, ου μονον τῳ εκδυομενον το γηρας νεαζειν, αλλα και αυξησιν επιδεχεσθαι μειζονα πεφυκε. και επειδαν το ὡρισμενον μετρον πληρωσῃ, εις ἑαυτον αναλισκεται. ὡς εν ταις ἱεραις ὁμοιως αυτος ὁ Taautos κατεταξε γραφαις. διο και εν ἱεροις τουτο το ζωον και εν μυστηριοις συμπαρειληπται.

spiral course, and at what degree of swiftness it pleases. And it is very long-lived, and has the quality not only of putting off its old age, and assuming a second youth, but it receives a greater increase. And when it has fulfilled the appointed measure of its existence, it consumes itself: as Taautus has laid down in the sacred books, wherefore this animal is introduced in the sacred rites and mysteries.—*Euseb. Præp. Evan.* lib. I. c. 10.

# THE FRAGMENTS

OF

# THE CHALDÆAN HISTORY:

FROM

BEROSSUS, ABYDENUS, AND MEGASTHENES.

# BEROSSUS:

## FROM APOLLODORUS.

### OF THE CHALDÆAN KINGS.

ΤΑΥΤΑ μεν ὁ Βηρωσσος ἱστορησε. Πρωτον γενεσθαι βασιλεα Αλωρον εκ Βαβυλωνος Χαλδαιον. βασιλευσαι δε σαρους δεκα. και καθεξης Αλαπαρον και Αμηλωνα τον εκ Παντιβιβλων. ειτα Αμμενωνα τον Χαλδαιον, εφ' οὑ (φησι) φανηναι τον μυσαρον Ωαννην τον Αννηδωτον εκ της Ερυθρας. (ὁπὲρ Αλεξανδρος προλαβων ειρηκε φανηναι τῳ πρωτῳ ετει. οὑτος δε μετα σαρους τεσσαρακοντα. ὁ δε Αβυδινος τον δευτερον Αννηδωτον μετα σαρους εικοσι ἑξ.) ειτα Μεγαλαρον εκ Παντιβιβλων πολεως. βασιλευσαι δε αυτον σαρους οκτωκαιδεκα. και μετα τουτον Δαωνον ποιμενα εκ Παντιβιβλων βασιλευσαι σαρους δεκα. κατα τουτον παλιν (φησι) φανηναι εκ της Ερυθρας Αννηδωτον τεταρτον την αυτην τοις ανω

THIS is the history which Berossus has transmitted to us. He tells us that the first king was Alorus of Babylon, a Chaldæan; he reigned ten sari: and afterwards Alaparus, and Amelon who came from Pantibiblon: then Ammenon the Chaldæan, in whose time appeared the Musarus Oannes the Annedotus from the Erythræan sea. (But Alexander Polyhistor anticipating the event, has said that he appeared in the first year; but Apollodorus says that it was after forty sari; Abydenus, however, makes the second Annedotus appear after twenty-six sari.) Then succeeded Megalarus from the city of Pantibiblon; and he reigned eighteen sari: and after him Daonus the shepherd from Pantibiblon reigned ten sari; in his time (he says) appeared again from the Erythræan sea a fourth Annedotus, having the same form with those above, the shape of εχοντα διαθεσιν, και την ιχθυος προς ανθρωπους μιξιν. ειτα ηρξαι Ευεδωρεσχον εκ Παντιβιβλων, και βασιλευσαι σαρους οκτωκαιδεκα. επι τουτου (φησιν) αλλον φανηναι εκ της Ερυθρας θαλασσης ὁμοιον κατα την ιχθυος προς ανθρωπον μιξιν, ᾧ ονομα Ωδακων. (Τουτους δε φησι παντας τα ὑπο Ωαννου κεφαλαιωδως ῥηθεντα κατα μερος εξηγησασθαι. περι τουτων Αβυδηνος ουδεν ειπεν.) ειτα αρξαι Αμεμψινον Χαλδαιον εκ Λαραγχων. βασιλευσαι δε αυτον ογδοον σαρους δεκα. ειτα αρξαι Ωτιαρτην Χαλδαιον εκ Λαραγχων. βασιλευσαι δε σαρους η΄. Ωτιαρτου δε τελευτησαντος τον υἱον αυτου Ξισουθρον βασιλευσαι σαρους οκτωκαιδεκα. επι τουτου τον μεγαν κατακλυσμον (φησι) γεγενησθαι. ὡς γινεσθαι ὁμου παντας βασιλεις δεκα· σαρους δε ἑκατον εικοσι.

a fish blended with that of a man. Then reigned Euedoreschus from Pantibiblon, for the term of eighteen sari; in his days there appeared another personage from the Erythræan sea like the former, having the same complicated form between a fish and a man, whose name was Odacon. (All these, says Apollodorus, related particularly and circumstantially whatever Oannes had informed them of: concerning these Abydenus has made no mention.) Then reigned Amempsinus, a Chaldæan from Laranchæ; and he being the eighth in order reigned ten sari. Then reigned Otiartes, a Chaldæan, from Laranchæ; and he reigned eight sari. And upon the death of Otiartes, his son Xisuthrus reigned eighteen sari: in his time happened the great deluge. So that the sum of all the kings is ten; and the term which they collectively reigned an hundred and twenty sari.—*Syncel. Chron.* 39. *Euseb. Chron.* 5.

# BEROSSUS:

## FROM ABYDENUS.

### OF THE CHALDÆAN KINGS AND THE DELUGE.

ΧΑΛΔΑΙΩΝ μεν της σοφιης περι τοσαυτα.

So much concerning the wisdom of the Chaldæans.

Βασιλευσαι δε της χωρας πρωτον λεγει Αλωρον. τον δε ὑπερ ἑαϋτου λογον διαδουναι, ὁτι μιν του λεω ποιμενα ὁ Θεος αποδειξαι. βασιλευσαι δε σαρους δεκα. σαρος δε εστι ἑξακοσια και τρισχιλια ετεα· νηρος δε ἑξακοσια· σωσσος δε εξηκοντα.

It is said that the first king of the country was Alorus, who gave out a report that he was appointed by God to be the Shepherd of the people: he reigned ten sari: now a sarus is esteemed to be three thousand six hundred years; a neros six hundred; and a sossus sixty.

Μετα δε τουτον Αλαπαρον αρξαι σαρους τρεις, μεθ' ὁν Αμιλλαρος εκ πολεως Παντιβιβλιος εβασιλευσεν σαρους ιγ'. εφ' οὗ δευτερον Αννηδωτον την θαλασσαν αναδυναι παραπλησιον Ωαννη την ιδεαν ἡμιδαιμονα. μεθ' ὁν Αμμενων εκ Παντιβιβλων ηρξε σαρους ιβ'. μεθ' ὁν Μεγαλαρος εκ Παντιβιβλων ηρξε σαρους οκτωκαιδεκα. ειτα Δαως ποιμην εκ Παντιβιβλων εβασιλευσεν

After him Alaparus reigned three sari: to him succeeded Amillarus from the city of Pantibiblon, who reigned thirteen sari; in his time a semidæmon called Annedotus, very like to Oannes, came up a second time from the sea: after him Ammenon reigned twelve sari, who was of the city of Pantibiblon: then Megalarus of the same place eighteen sari: then Daos, the shepherd, governed for the space of ten sari; he was of Pantibiblon; in his time σαρους δεκα, εφ᾽ ού δ᾽ διφυεις γην εκ θαλασσης ανεδυσαν, ὥντα ονομαῖα ταυῖα· Ευεδωκος, Ενευγαμος, Ενευβουλος, Ανημεντος. επι δε του μετα ταυτα Ευεδωρεσχου Ανωδαφος· μεθ᾽ ὅυς αλλοιτε ηρξαν, και Σεισιθρος επι τουτοις. ώς τους παντας ειναι βασιλεις δεκα· ὧν ὁ χρονος της βασιλειας συνηρξε σαρους ἑκατον εικοσι. (και περι του κατακλυσμου, παρ᾽ ὁμοια μεν ουκ απαραλλακτα λεγει οὕτως.) μετ᾽ Ευεδωρεσχον αλλοι τινες ηρξαν και Σεισιθρος· ῳ̃ δη Κρονος προσημαινει μεν εσεσθαι πληθος ομβρων Δεσιου πεμπτη επι δεκα. κελευει δε παν ὁ,τι γραμματων ην εχομενον, εν ἡλιου πολει τῃ̃ εν Σιππαροισιν αποκρυψαι. Σεισιθρος δε ταυτα επιτελεα ποιησας, ευθεως επ᾽ Αρμενιους ανεπλωε, και παραυτικα μιν κατελαμβανε τα εκ θεου. Τριτῃ δε ἡμερῃ επειτα ὧν εκοπασε, μετηει των ορνιθων πειρην ποιευμενος, εικου γην ιδοιεν του ὕδατος εκδυσαν. Αἱ δε εκδεχομενου σφεας πελαγεος αχανεος, απορευσαι ὀκη καθορμηνται, παρα τον Σεισιθρον οπισω κομιζονται, και επ᾽ αυτησιν ἑτεραι. ῾Ως δε τῃσι τριτῃσι ευτυχεεν, απικατο γαρ δη πηλου καταπλεοι τους ταρ-

four double-shaped personages came out of the sea to land, whose names were Euedocus, Eneugamus, Eneuboulus, and Anementus: after these things was Anodaphus, in the time of Euedoreschus. There were afterwards other kings, and last of all Sisithrus: so that in the whole, the number amounted to ten kings, and the term of their reigns to an hundred and twenty sari. (And among other things not irrelative to the subject, he continues thus concerning the deluge:) After Euedoreschus some others reigned, and then Sisithrus. To him the deity Cronus foretold that on the fifteenth day of the month Desius there would be a deluge, and commanded him to deposit all the writings whatever that he had, in the city of the Sun in Sippara. Sisithrus, when he had complied with these commands, instantly sailed to Armenia, and was immediately inspired by God. During the prevalence of the waters Sisithrus sent out birds, that he might judge if the flood had subsided. But the birds passing over an unbounded sea, and not finding any place of rest, returned again to Sisithrus. This he repeated. And when upon the third trial he succeeded, for they then returned with their feet stained with mud, the gods translated him from among men. With respect to the vessel, which yet στους, θεοι μιν εξ ανθρωπων αφανιζουσιν. Το δε πλοιον εν Αρμενιη περιαττα ξυλων αλεξιφαρμακα τοισιν επιχωριοισι παρειχετο.

remains in Armenia, it is a custom of the inhabitants to form bracelets and amulets of its wood.—*Syncel.* 38. — *Euseb. Præp. Evan.* lib. 9. — *Euseb. Chron.* 5. 8.

## OF THE TOWER OF BABEL.

Εντι δ' οἱ λεγουσι τους πρωτους εκ γης ανασχοντας, ῥωμη τε και μεγεθει χαυνωθεντας, και δη θεων καταφρονησαντας, αμεινονας ειναι, πυργον τυρσιν ἠλιβατον αειρειν, ἱνα νυν Βαβυλων εστιν· ηδη τε ασσον ειναι του ουρανου. και τους ανεμους, θεοισι βωθεοντας ανατρεψαι περι αυτοισι το μηχανημα. του δητα ερειπια λεγεσθαι Βαβυλωνα. τεως δε οντας ὁμογλωσσους εκ θεων πολυθρα φωνην ενεικασθαι, μετα δε Κρονῳ τε και Τιτηνι συστηναι πολεμον. ὁ δε τοπος εν ᾡ πυργον ῳκοδομησαν, νυν Βαβυλων καλειται, δια την συγχυσιν του περι την διαλεκτον πρωτον εναργους. Ἑβραιοι γαρ την συγχυσιν Βαβελ καλουσι.

They say that the first inhabitants of the earth, glorying in their own strength and size, and despising the gods, undertook to raise a tower whose top should reach the sky, where Babylon now stands: but when it approached the heaven, the winds assisted the gods, and overturned the work upon its contrivers: and its ruins are said to be at Babylon: and the gods introduced a diversity of tongues among men, who till that time had all spoken the same language: and a war arose between Cronus and Titan: but the place in which they built the tower is now called Babylon, on account of the confusion of the tongues; for confusion is by the Hebrews called Babel. —*Euseb. Præp. Evan.* lib. 9.—*Syncel. Chron.* 44.—*Euseb. Chron.* 13.

# BEROSSUS:

## FROM ALEXANDER POLYHISTOR.

### OF THE COSMOGONY ~~AND CAUSES OF~~ THE DELUGE.

ΒΗΡΩΣΣΟΣ δε εν τη πρωτη των Βαβυλωνιακων φησι, γενεσθαι μεν αυτον κατα Αλεξανδρον τον Φιλιππου την ἡλικιαν. αναγραφας δε πολλων εν Βαβυλωνι φυλασσεσθαι μετα πολλης επιμελειας απο ετων που ὑπερ μυριαδων δεκαπεντε περιεχουσας χρονον· περιεχειν δε τας αναγραφας ἱστοριας περι του ουρανου, και θαλασσης, και πρωτογονιας, και βασιλεων, και των κατ' αυτους πραξεων.

BEROSSUS, in his first book concerning the history of Babylonia, informs us that he lived in the time of Alexander the son of Philip. And he mentions that there were written accounts preserved at Babylon with the greatest care, comprehending a term of fifteen myriads of years. These writings contained a history of the heavens and the sea; of the birth of mankind; also of those who had sovereign rule; and of the actions achieved by them.

Και πρωτον μεν την Βαβυλωνιαν γην (φησι) κεισθαι επι του Τιγριδος και Ευφρατου ποταμου μεσην. φυειν δε αυτην πυρους αγριους, και κριθας, και οχρον, και σησαμον, και τας εν τοις ἑλεσι φυομενας ῥιζας εσθιεσθαι ονομαζεσθαι αυτας γογγας· ισοδυναμειν δε τας ῥιζας

And in the first place he describes Babylonia as a country which lay between the Tigris and Euphrates. He mentions that it abounded with wheat, barley, ocrus, sesamum; and in the lakes were found the roots called gongæ, which were good to be eaten, and were in respect to nutriment like barley. There were also palm trees and apples, and most ταυτας κριθαις. γινεσθαι δε φοινικας, και μηλα, και τα λοιπα ακροδρυα, και ιχθυας και ορνεα, χερσαια τε και λιμναια. ειναι δε αυτης τα μεν κατα Αραβιαν μερη ανυδρα τε και ακαρπα. τα δε αντικειμενα τη Αραβια, ορεινα τε και ευφορα. εν δε τη Βαβυλωνι πολυ πληθος ανθρωπων γενεσθαι αλλοεθνων κατοικησαντων την Χαλδαιαν· ζην δε αυτους ατακτως, ώσπερ τα θηρια.

Εν δε τῳ πρωτῳ ενιαυτῳ φανηναι εκ της Ερυθρας θαλασσης κατα τον όμορουντα τοπον τη Βαβυλωνια ζωον αφρενον ονοματι Ωαννην, (καθως και Απολλοδωρος ἱστορησε,) το μεν όλον σωμα εχον ιχθυος· ὑπο δε την κεφαλην παραπεφυκυιαν αλλην κεφαλην ὑπο κατω της του ιχθυος κεφαλης, και ποδας ὁμοιως ανθρωπου, παραπεφυκοτας δε εκ της ουρας του ιχθυος· ειναι δε αυτῳ φωνην ανθρωπου, την δε εικονα αυτου ετι και νυν διαφυλασσεσθαι.

Τουτο δε (φησιν) το ζωον την μεν ἡμεραν διατριβειν μετα των ανθρωπων, μηδεμιαν τροφην προσφερομενον· παραδιδοναι τε τοις ανθρωποις γραμματων, και μαθηματων, και τεχνων παντοδαπων εμπειριαν, και πολεων συνοικισμους, και ἱερων

kinds of fruits; fish too and birds; both those which are merely of flight, and those which take to the element of water. The part of Babylonia which is bordered upon Arabia, was barren, and without water; but that which lay on the other side had hills, and was fruitful. At Babylon there was (in these times) a great resort of people of various nations, who inhabited Chaldea, and lived without rule and order like the beast of the field.

In the first year there made its appearance, from a part of the Erythræan sea which bordered upon Babylonia, an animal endowed with reason, who was called Oannes. (According to the account of Apollodorus) the whole body of the animal was like that of a fish; and had under a fish's head another head, and also feet below, similar to those of a man, subjoined to the fish's tail. His voice too, and language, was articulate and human; and a representation of him is preserved even to this day.

This Being in the day-time used to converse with men; but took no food at that season; and he gave them an insight into letters and sciences, and every kind of art. He taught them to construct houses, to found temples, to compile laws, and explained to them the principles of ἱδρυσεις, και νομων εισηγησεις, και γεωμετριαν διδασκειν, και σπερματα, και καρπων συναγωγας ὑποδεικνυειν, και συνολως παντα τα προς ἡμερωσιν ανηκοντα βιου παραδιδοναι τοις ανθρωποις. απο δε του χρονου εκεινου ουδεν αλλο περισσον εὑρεθηναι. του δε ἡλιου δυναντος το ζωον τουτον Ωαννην δυναι παλιν εις την θαλατταν, και τας νυκτας εκει διαιτασθαι· ειναι γαρ αυτον αμφιβιον.

Ὑστερον δε φανηναι και ἑτερα ζωα ὁμοια τουτων, περι ὡν εν τῃ των βασιλεων αναγραφῃ (φησιν) δηλωσειν.

Τον δε Ωαννην περι γενεας και πολιτειας γραψαι, και παραδουναι τονδε τον λογον τοις ανθρωποις.

"Γενεσθαι" φησι "χρονον, εν ᾧ το παν σκοτος και ὑδωρ ειναι, και εν τουτοις ζωα τερατωδη, και ειδιφυεις τας ιδεας εχοντα ζωογονεισθαι. ανθρωπους γαρ διπτερους γεννηθηναι, ενιους δε και τετραπτερους, και διπροσωπους· και σωμα μεν εχοντας ἑν, κεφαλας δε δυο, ανδρειαν τε και γυναικειαν, και αιδοια τε διττα, αρρεν και θηλυ· και ἑτερους ανθρωπους, τους μεν αιγων σκελη και κερατα εχοντας, τους δε ἱππο-

geometrical knowledge. He made them distinguish the seeds of the earth, and shewed them how to collect fruits; in short, he instructed them in every thing which could tend to soften manners and humanize mankind. From that time, so universal were his instructions, nothing has been added material by way of improvement. When the sun set, it was the custom of this Being to plunge again into the sea, and abide all night in the deep; for he was amphibious.

After this there appeared other animals like Oannes, of which Berossus promises to give an account when he comes to the history of the kings.

Moreover Oannes wrote concerning the generation of mankind; of their different ways of life, and of their civil polity; and the following is the purport of what he said:

"There was a time in which there was nothing but darkness and an abyss of waters, wherein resided most hideous beings, which were produced of a two-fold principle. Men appeared with two wings, some with four and with two faces. They had one body but two heads; the one of a man, the other of a woman. They were likewise in their several organs both male and female. Other human figures were to be seen with the legs and horns of goats. Some had horses' feet: others had the limbs of a horse ποδας, τας δε τα οπισω μεν μερη ἱππων, τα δε εμπροσθεν ανθρωπων, οἱς ἱπποκενταυρους την ιδεαν ειναι. ζωογονηθηναι δε και ταυρους ανθρωπων κεφαλας εχοντας· και κυνας τετρασωματους, ουρας ιχθυος εκ των οπισθεν μερων εχοντας, και ἱππους κυνοκεφαλους, και ανθρωπους, και ἑτερα ζωα κεφαλας μεν και σωματα ἱππων εχοντα, ουρας δε ιχθυων. και αλλα δε ζωα παντοδαπων θηριων μορφας εχοντα. προς δε τουτοις, ιχθυας, και ἑρπετα, και οφεις, και αλλα ζωα πλειονα θαυμαστα και παρηλλαγμενα τας οψεις αλληλων εχοντα· ὡν και τας εικονας εν τῳ του Βηλου ναῳ ανακεισθαι.

behind, but before were fashioned like men, resembling hippocentaurs. Bulls likewise bred there with the heads of men; and dogs with fourfold bodies, and the tails of fishes. Also horses with the heads of dogs: men too and other animals, with the heads and bodies of horses and the tails of fishes. In short, there were creatures with the limbs of every species of animals. Add to these fishes, reptiles, serpents, with other wonderful animals, which assumed each other's shape and countenance. Of all these were preserved delineations in the temple of Belus at Babylon.

"Αρχειν δε τουτων παντων γυναικα ᾗ ονομα Ομορωκα· ειναι δε τουτο Χαλδαϊστι μεν Θαλατθ, Ἑλληνιστι δε μεθερμηνευεται θαλασσα, κατα δε ισοψηφον σεληνη· οὑτως δε των ὁλων συνεστηκοτων, επανελθοντα Βηλον σχισαι την γυναικα μεσην, και το μεν ἡμισυ αυτης ποιησαι γην, το δε αλλο ἡμισυ ουρανον, και τα ἐν αυτῃ ζωα αφανισαι. αλληγορικως δε (φησιν) τουτο μεν φυσιολογεισθαι. ὑγρου γαρ οντος του παντος, και ζωων εν αυτῳ γεγεννημενων, τουτον τον

"The person, who was supposed to have presided over them, was a woman named Omoroca; which in the Chaldaic language is Thalatth; which the Greeks express Thalassa, the sea: but according to the most true computation, it is equivalent to Selene, the moon. All things being in this situation, Belus came, and cut the woman asunder: and out of one half of her he formed the earth, and of the other half the heavens; and at the same time destroyed the animals in the abyss. All this (he says) was an allegorical description of nature. For the whole universe consisting of

Θεων αφελειν την ἑαυτου κεφαλην, και το ῥυεν αἱμα τους αλλους θεους φυρασθαι τη γη, και διαπλασαι τους ανθρωπους· δια νοερους τε ειναι, και φρονησεως θειας μετεχειν. τον δε Βηλον, ὁν Δια μεθερμηνευουσι, μεσον τεμοντα το σκοτος χωρισαι γην και ουρανον απ' αλληλων, και διαταξαι τον κοσμον· τα δε ζωα ουκ ενεγκοντα την του φωτος δυναμιν φθαρηναι. ιδοντα δε τον Βηλον χωραν ερημον και καρποφορον, κελευσαι ἑνι των θεων την κεφαλην αφελοντι ἑαυτου τῳ απορῥυεντι αἱματι φυρασαι την γην, και διαπλασαι ανθρωπους, και θηρια τα δυναμενα τον αερα φερειν· αποτελεσαι δε τον Βηλον, και αστρα, και ἡλιον, και σεληνην, και τους πεντε πλανητας."

moisture, and animals being continually generated therein; the deity (Belus) above-mentioned cut off his own head: upon which the other gods mixed the blood, as it gushed out, with the earth; and from thence men were formed. On this account it is that they are rational, and partake of divine knowledge. This Belus, whom men call Dis, divided the darkness, and separated the Heavens from the Earth, and reduced the universe to order. But the animals so lately created, not being able to bear the prevalence of light, died. Belus upon this, seeing a vast space quite uninhabited, though by nature very fruitful, ordered one of the gods to take off his head; and when it was taken off, they were to mix the blood with the soil of the earth; and from thence to form other men and animals, which should be capable of bearing the light. Belus also formed the stars, and the sun, and the moon, together with the five planets.

(Εν δε τη δευτερᾳ τους δεκα βασιλεις των Χαλδαιων, και τον χρονον της βασιλειας αυτων, σαρους ἑκατον εικοσι, ητοι ετων μυριαδας τεσσαρακοντα τρεις, και δυο χιλιαδας, ἑως του κατακλυσμου. λεγει γαρ ὁ αυτος Αλεξανδρος, ὡς απο της γραφης των Χαλδαιων αυθις παρακατιων απο εννατου

(In the second book was the history of the ten kings of the Chaldeans, and the periods of each reign, which consisted collectively of an hundred and twenty sari, or four hundred and thirty-two thousand years; reaching to the time of the Deluge. For Alexander, as from the writings of the Chaldæans, enumerating the kings from the ninth Ardates to Xisuthrus, βασιλεως Αρδατου επι τον δεκατον λεγομενον παρ' αυτοις Ξισουθρον, ούτως.)

Αρδατου δε τελευτησαντος τον υἱον αυτου Ξισουθρον βασιλευσαι σαρους οκτωκαιδεκα· επι τουτου μεγαν κατακλυσμον γενεσθαι. αναγεγραφθαι δε τον λογον ούτως. τον Κρονον αυτῳ κατα τον ὑπνον επισταντα φαναι, μηνος Δαισια πεμπτῃ και δεκατῃ τους ανθρωπους ὑπο κατακλυσμου φθαρησεσθαι. κελευσαι ουν δια γραμματων παντων αρχας και μεσα και τελετας ορυξαντα θειναι εν πολει ἡλιου Σιππαροις, και ναυπηγησαμενον σκαφος εμβηναι μετα των συγγενων και αναγκαιων φιλων· ενθεσθαι δε βρωματα και πωματα, εμβαλειν δε και ζωα πτηνα και τετραποδα, και παντα ευτρεπισαμενον, πλειν. ερωτωμενον δε που πλει; φαναι, προς τους Θεους· ευξαμενον ανθρωποις αγαθα γενεσθαι. τον δ' ου παρακουσαντα, ναυπηγησαντα σκαφος, το μεν μηκος σταδιων πεντε, το δε πλατος σταδιων δυο· τα δε συνταχθεντα παντα συνθεσθαι, και γυναικα, και τεκνα, και τους αναγκαιους φιλους εμβιβασαι. γενομενου δε του κατακλυσμου, και ευθεως ληξαντος· των ορνεων τινα

who is called by them the tenth, proceeds in this manner:)

After the death of Ardates, his son Xisuthrus succeeded, and reigned eighteen sari. In his time happened the great Deluge; the history of which is given in this manner. The Deity, Cronus, appeared to him in a vision, and gave him notice that upon the fifteenth day of the month Dæsia there would be a flood, by which mankind would be destroyed. He therefore enjoined him to commit to writing a history of the beginning, procedure, and final conclusion of all things, down to the present term; and to bury these accounts securely in the city of the Sun at Sippara; and to build a vessel, and to take with him into it his friends and relations; and to convey on board every thing necessary to sustain life, and to take in also all species of animals, that either fly or rove upon the earth; and trust himself to the deep. Having asked the Deity, whither he was to sail? he was answered, "To the Gods:" upon which he offered up a prayer for the good of mankind. And he obeyed the divine admonition: and built a vessel five stadia in length, and in breadth two. Into this he put every thing which he had got ready; and last of all conveyed into it his wife, τον Ξισουθρον αφιεναι. τα δε ου τροφην εὑροντα ουτε τοπον ὁπου καθισαι, παλιν ελθειν εις το πλοιον. τον δε Ξισουθρον παλιν μετα τινας ἡμερας αφιεναι τα ορνεα· ταυτα δε παλιν εις την ναυν ελθειν τους ποδας πεπηλαμενους εχοντα· το δε τριτον αφεθεντα, ουκ ετι ελθειν εις το πλοιον. τον δε Ξισουθρον εννοηθηναι γην αναπεφηνεναι· διελοντα τε των του πλοιου ῥαφων μερος τι, και ιδοντα προσοκειλαν το πλοιον ορει τινι, εκβηναι μετα της γυναικος, και της θυγατρος, και του κυβερνητου· προσκυνησαντα την γην, και βωμον ἱδρυσαμενον, και θυσιασαντα τοις θεοις, γενεσθαι μετα των εκβαντων του πλοιου αφανη. τους δε ὑπομειναντας εν τῳ πλοιῳ, μη εισπορευομενων των περι τον Ξισουθρον, εκβαντας ζητειν αυτον επι ονοματος βοωντας. τον δε Ξισουθρον αυτον μεν αυτοις ουκ ετι οφθηναι· φωνην δε εκ του αερος γενεσθαι, κελευουσαν, ὡς δεον αυτους ειναι θεοσεβεις, και παρ' αυτων δια την ευσεβειαν πορευεσθαι μετα των θεων οικησοντα. της δε αυτης τιμης και την γυναικα αυτου, και την θυγατερα, και τον κυβερνητην μετεσχηκεναι. ειπεν τε

children, and friends. After the flood had been upon the earth, and was in time abated, Xisuthrus sent out some birds from the vessel; which not finding any food, nor any place to rest their feet, returned to him again. After an interval of some days, he sent them forth a second time; and they now returned with their feet tinged with mud. He made a trial a third time with these birds; but they returned to him no more: from whence he formed a judgment, that the surface of the earth was now above the waters. Having therefore made an opening in the vessel, and finding upon looking out, that the vessel was driven to the side of a mountain, he immediately quitted it, being attended by his wife, his daughter, and the pilot. Xisuthrus immediately paid his adoration to the earth: and having constructed an altar, offered sacrifices to the gods. These things being duly performed, both Xisuthrus and those who came out of the vessel with him, disappeared. They, who remained in the vessel, finding that the others did not return, came out with many lamentations, and called continually on the name of Xisuthrus. Him they saw no more; but they could distinguish his voice in the air, and could hear him admonish them to pay due regard to the gods; and likewise αυτοις· ὁτι ελευσονται παλιν εις Βαβυλωνα, και ὡς ειμαρται αυτοις, εκ Σιππαρων ανελομενοις τα γραμματα διαδουναι τοις ανθρωποις· και ὁτι ὁπου εισιν, ἡ χωρα Αρμενιας εστιν· τους δε ακουσαντας ταυτα θυσαι τε τοις θεοις, και περιξι πορευθηναι εις Βαβυλωνα.

inform them that it was upon account of his piety that he was translated to live with the gods; that his wife and daughter, with the pilot, had obtained the same honour. To this he added that he would have them make the best of their way to Babylonia, and search for the writings at Sippara, which were to be made known to all mankind: and that the place where they then were was the land of Armenia. The remainder having heard these words, offered sacrifices to the gods; and taking a circuit, journeyed towards Babylonia.

Του δε πλοιου τουτου κατακλασθεντος εν τῃ Αρμενιᾳ ετι μερος τι αυτου εν τοις Κορκυραιων ορεσι της Αρμενιας διαμενειν, και τινας απο του πλοιου κομιζειν αποξυοντας ασφαλτον, χρασθαι δε αυτην προς τους αποτροπιασμους. ελθοντας ουν τουτους εις Βαβυλωνα, τα τε εκ Σιππαρων γραμματα ανορυξαι, και πολεις πολλας κτιζοντας, και ἱερα ανιδρυσαμενους, παλιν επικτισαι την Βαβυλωνα.

The vessel being thus stranded in Armenia, some part of it yet remains in the Corcyræan mountains in Armenia; and the people scrape off the bitumen, with which it had been outwardly coated, and make use of it by way of an alexipharmic and amulet. In this manner they returned to Babylon; and having found the writings at Sippara, they set about building cities, and erecting temples: and Babylon was thus inhabited again.—*Syncel. Chron.* 28.—*Euseb. Chron.* 5. 8.

## OF ABRAHAM.

Μετα τον κατακλυσμον δεκατῃ γενεᾳ, παρα Χαλδαιοις τις ην δικαιος ανηρ, και μεγας, και τα ουρανια εμπειρος.

After the deluge, in the tenth genertion, was a certain man among the Chaldæans renowned for his justice and great exploits, and for his skill in the celestial sciences. — *Euseb. Præp. Evan.* lib. 9.

## OF NABONASAR.

Απο δε Ναβονασαρου τους χρονους της των αστερων κινησεως Χαλδαιοι ηκριβωσαν, και απο Χαλδαιων οἱ παρ' Ἑλλησι μαθηματικοι λαβοντες· πειδαν Ναβονασαρος συναγαγων τας πραξεις των προ αυτου βασιλεων, ηφανισεν, ὁπως απ' αυτου ἡ καταριθμησις γινεται των Χαλδαιων βασιλεων.

From the reign of Nabonasar only are the Chaldæans (from whom the Greek mathematicians copy) accurately acquainted with the heavenly motions: for Nabonasar collected all the mementos of the kings prior to himself, and destroyed them, that the enumeration of the Chaldæan kings might commence with him.— *Syncel. Chron.* 207.

## OF THE DESTRUCTION OF THE JEWISH TEMPLE.

Τινα τροπον πεμψας επι την Αιγυπτον και επι την ἡμετεραν γην τον υἱον τον ἑαυτου Ναβουχοδονοσορον μετα πολλης δυναμεως, επειδηπερ αφεστατας αυτους επυθετο, παντων εκρατησε, και τον ναον ενεπρησε τον εν Ἱεροσολυμοις,

He (Nabopollasar) sent his son Nabuchodonosor with a great army against Egypt, and against Judea, upon his being informed that they had revolted from him; and by that means he subdued them all, and set fire to the temple that was at Jerusalem; and removed our people entirely out ὅλας τε παντα τον παρ' ἡμιν λαον αναστησας, εις Βαβυλωνα μετῳκισεν. συνεβη δε και την πολιν ερημωθηναι χρονον ετων ἑβδομηκοντα, μεχρι Κυρου του Περσων βασιλεως. κρατησαι δε (φησι) τον Βαβυλωνιον Αιγυπτου, Συριας, Φοινικης, Αραβιας, παντας δε ὑπερβαλλομενον ταις πραξεσι τους προ αυτου Χαλδαιων και Βαβυλωνιων βεβασιλευκοτας.

of their own country, and transferred them to Babylon, and it happened that our city was desolate during the interval of seventy years, until the days of Cyrus king of Persia. (He then says, that) this Babylonian king conquered Egypt, and Syria, and Phœnicia, and Arabia, and exceeded in his exploits all that had reigned before him in Babylon and Chaldæa. — *Joseph. contr. Appion.* lib. I. c. 19.

## OF NEBUCHADNEZZAR.

Ακουσας δε ὁ πατηρ αυτου Ναβοπολλασαρος, ὁτι ὁ τεταγμενος σατραπης εν τε Αιγυπτῳ και τοις περι την Συριαν την Κοιλην και την Φοινικην τοποις αποστατης γεγονεν, ου δυναμενος αυτος ετι κακοπαθειν, συστησας τῳ υἱῳ Ναβουχοδονοσορῳ οντι ετι εν ἡλικιᾳ μερη τινα της δυναμεως εξεπεμψεν επ' αυτον. συμμιξας δε Ναβουχοδονοσορος τῳ αποστατῃ, και παραταξαμενος αυτου τε εκυριευσεν, και την χωραν εξ αρχης ὑπο την αὑτου βασιλειαν εποιησεν. τῳ δε πατρι αυτου συνεβη Ναβοπολλασαρῳ κατα τουτον τον καιρον αρρωστησαντι, εν τῃ Βαβυλωνιων πολει μεταλλαξαι τον βιον, ετη βεβασιλευκοτι εικοσιν εννεα.

When Nabopollasar his (Nabuchodonosor's) father, heard that the governor, whom he had set over Egypt, and the parts of Cœlesyria and Phœnicia, had revolted, he was unable to put up with his delinquencies any longer, but committed certain parts of his army to his son Nabuchodonosor, who was then but young, and sent him against the rebel: and Nabuchodonosor fought with him, and conquered him, and reduced the country again under his dominion. And it happened that his father, Nabopollasar, fell into a distemper at this time, and died in the city of Babylon, after he had reigned twenty-nine years.

Αισθομενος δε μετ' ου πολυ την του πατρος τελευτην Ναβουχοδονοσορος, καταστησας τα κατα την Αιγυπτον πραγματα και την λοιπην χωραν, και τους αιχμαλωτους Ιουδαιων τε και Φοινικων και Συρων και των κατα την Αιγυπτον εθνων συνταξας τισι των φιλων, μετα βαρυτατης δυναμεως και της λοιπης ωφελειας ανακομιζειν εις την Βαβυλωνιαν, αυτος ὁρμησας ὀλιγοστος παρεγενετο δια της ερημου εις Βαβυλωνα. καταλαβων δε τα πραγματα διοικουμενα ὑπο Χαλδαιων, και διατηρουμενην την βασιλειαν ὑπο του βελτιστου αυτων, κυριευσας εξ ὁλοκληρου της πατρικης αρχης, τοις μεν αιχμαλωτοις παραγενομενοις συνεταξεν αυτοις αποικιας εν τοις επιτηδειοτατοις της Βαβυλωνιας τοπους αποδειξαι· αυτος δε απο των εκ του πολεμου λαφυρων, τοτε Βηλου ἱερον και τα λοιπα κοσμησας φιλοτιμως, την τε ὑπαρχουσαν εξ αρχης πολιν, και ἑτεραν εξωθεν προσχαρισαμενος και ανακαινισας, προς το μηκετι δυνασθαι τους πολιορκουντας τον ποταμον αναστρεφοντας επι την πολιν κατασκευαζειν, ὑπερεβαλετο τρεις μεν της ενδον πολεως περιβολους, τρεις δε της εξω

After a short time Nabuchodonosor, receiving the intelligence of his father's death, set the affairs of Egypt and the other countries, in order, and committed the captives he had taken from the Jews, and Phœnicians, and Syrians, and of the nations belonging to Egypt, to some of his friends, that they might conduct that part of the forces that had on heavy armour, with the rest of his baggage, to Babylonia; while he went in haste, with a few followers, across the desert to Babylon; where, when he was come, he found that affairs had been well conducted by the Chaldæans, and that the principal person among them had preserved the kingdom for him: accordingly he now obtained possession of all his father's dominions. And he ordered the captives to be distributed in colonies in the most proper places of Babylonia: and adorned the temple of Belus, and the other temples, in a sumptuous and pious manner, out of the spoils he had taken in this war. He also rebuilt the old city, and added another to it on the outside, and so far restored Babylon, that none, who should besiege it afterwards, might have it in their power to divert the river, so as to facilitate an entrance into it: and this he did by building three walls about the inner city, and three about the outer. Some of these walls he τουτων, τους μεν εξ οπτης πλινθου και ασφαλτου, τους δε εξ αυτης της πλινθου. και τειχισας αξιολογως την πολιν, και τους πυλωνας κοσμησας ἱεροπρεπως, προσκατεσκευακεν τοις πατρικοις βασιλειοις ἑτερα βασιλεια εχομενα εκεινων, ὑπεραιροντα αναστημα και την πολλην πολυτελειαν. μακρα δ' ισως εσται εαν τις εξηγηται, πλην οντα γε εις ὑπερβολην ὡς μεγαλα και ὑπερηφανα, συνετελεσθη ἡμεραις δεκαπεντε. εν δε τοις βασιλειοις τουτοις αναλημματα λιθινα ὑψηλα ανῳκοδομησας, και την οψιν αποδους ὁμοιοτατην τοις ορεσι, καταφυτευσας δενδρεσι παντοδαποις εξειργασατο, και κατασκευασας τον καλουμενον κρεμαστον παραδεισον, δια το την γυναικα αυτου επιθυμειν της ορειας διαθεσεως, τεθραμμενην εν τοις κατα την Μηδιαν τοποις.

built of burnt brick and bitumen, and some of brick only. When he had thus admirably fortified the city with walls, and had magnificently adorned the gates, he added also a new palace to those in which his forefathers had dwelt, adjoining them, but exceeding them in height, and in its great splendor. It would perhaps require too long a narration, if any one were to describe it: however, as prodigiously large and magnificent as it was, it was finished in fifteen days. In this palace he erected very high walks, supported by stone pillars; and by planting what was called a pensile paradise, and replenishing it with all sorts of trees, he rendered the prospect an exact resemblance of a mountainous country. This he did to please his queen, because she had been brought up in Media, and was fond of a mountainous situation. —*Joseph. contr. Appion.* lib. 1. c. 19. —*Syncel. Chron.* 220.—*Euseb. Præp. Evan.* lib. 9.

## OF THE CHALDÆAN KINGS AFTER NEBUCHADNEZZAR.

Ναβουχοδονοσορος μεν ουν μετα το αρξασθαι του προειρημενου τειχους, εμπεσων εις αρρωστιαν, μετηλλαξατο τον βιον, βεβασιλευκως ετη τεσ-

Nabuchodonosor, after he had begun to build the abovementioned wall, fell sick, and departed this life, when he had reigned forty-three years; whereupon his son Evilmerodachus *σαρακονταττρια. της δε βασιλειας κυριος εγενετο ὁ υἱος αυτου Ευειλμαραδουχος. οὑτος προστας των πραγματων ανομως και ασελγως, επιβουλευθεις ὑπο του την αδελφην εχοντος αυτου Νηριγλισσοορου αιηρεθη, βασιλευσας ετη δυο.*

*Μετα δε το αναιρεθηναι τουτον, διαδεξαμενος την αρχην ὁ επιβουλευσας αυτῳ Νηριγλισσοορος, εβασιλευσεν ετη τεσσαρα.*

*Τουτου υἱος Λαβοροσοαρχοδος εκυριευσε μεν της βασιλειας παις ων μηνας εννεα· επιβουλευθεις δε, δια το πολλα εμφαινειν κακοηθη, ὑπο των φιλων απετυμπανισθη.*

*Απολομενου δε τουτου, συνελθοντες οἱ επιβουλευσαντες αυτῳ, κοινῃ την βασιλειαν περιεθηκαν Ναβοννηδῳ τινι των εκ Βαβυλωνος, οντι εκ της αυτης επισυστασεως. επι τουτου τα περι του ποταμου τειχη της Βαβυλωνιων πολεως, εξ οπτης πλινθου και ασφαλτου κατεκοσμηθη.*

*Ουσης δε της βασιλειας αυτου εν τῳ ἑπτακαιδεκατῳ ετει, προεξεληλυθως Κυρος εκ της Περσιδος μετα δυναμεως πολλης, και καταστρεψαμενος την λοιπην Ασιαν πασαν, ὡρ-*

obtained the kingdom. He governed public affairs in an illegal and improper manner, and by means of a plot laid against him by Neriglissoorus, his sister's husband, was slain when he had reigned but two years.

After his death Neriglissoorus, who had conspired against him, succeeded him in the kingdom, and reigned four years.

His son Laborosoarchodus obtained the kingdom though he was but a child, and kept it nine months; but by reason of the evil practices he exhibited, a plot was laid against him by his friends, and he was tormented to death.

After his death, the conspirators assembled, and by common consent put the crown upon the head of Nabonnedus, a man of Babylon, and one of the leaders of that insurrection. In his reign it was that the walls of the city of Babylon were curiously built with burnt brick and bitumen.

But in the seventeenth year of his reign, Cyrus came out of Persia with a great army, and having conquered all the rest of Asia, he came hastily to Babylonia. When Nabonnedus perceived he was advancing to atμησεν επι της Βαβυλωνος· αισθομενος δε Ναβοννηδος την εφοδον αυτου, απαντησας μετα της δυναμεως και παραταξαμενος, ἡττηθεις τη μαχη και φυγων ολιγοστος, συνεκλεισθη εις την Βορσιππηνων πολιν. Κυρος δε Βαβυλωνα καταλαβομενος, και συνταξας τα εξω της πολεως τειχη κατασκαψαι, δια το λιαν αυτῳ πραγματικην και δυσαλωτον φανηναι την πολιν, ανεζευξεν επι Βορσιππον, εκπολιορκησων τον Ναβοννηδον. του δε Ναβοννηδου ουχ ὑπομειναντος την πολιορκιαν, ἀλλ' εγχειρισαντος αὑτον, προτερον χρησαμενος Κυρος φιλανθρωπως, και δους οικητηριον αυτῳ Καρμανιαν, εξεπεμψεν εκ της Βαβυλωνιας. Ναβοννηδος μεν ουν το λοιπον του χρονου διαγενομενος εν εκεινη τη χωρᾳ, κατεστρεψε τον βιον.

tack him, he assembled his forces and opposed him, but was defeated, and fled with a few of his attendants, and was shut up in the city Borsippus. Whereupon Cyrus took Babylon, and gave orders that the outer walls should be demolished, because the city had proved very troublesome to him, and difficult to take. He then marched to Borsippus, to besiege Nabonnedus; but as Nabonnedus delivered himself into his hands without holding out the place, he was at first kindly treated by Cyrus, who gave him an habitation in Carmania, but sent him out of Babylonia. Accordingly Nabonnedus spent the remainder of his time in that country, and there died.—*Joseph. contr. App.* lib. 1. c. 20.—*Euseb. Præp. Evan.* lib. 10.

## OF THE FEAST OF SACEA.

Βηρωσσος δε εν πρωτῳ Βαβυλωνιακων, τῳ Λῳῳ, φησι, μηνι εκκαιδεκατῃ αγεσθαι ἑορτην Σακεας προσαγορευομενην εν Βαβυλωνι επι ἡμερας πεντε, εν αἱς εθος ειναι αρχεσθαι τους δεσποτας ὑπο των οικετων,

Berossus, in the first book of his Babylonian history, says; That in the eleventh month, called Loos, is celebrated in Babylon the feast of Sacea for five days; in which it is the custom that the masters should obey their domestics, one of whom is led αφηγεισθαι τε της οικιας ἑνα αυτων ενδεδυκοτα στολην ὁμοιαν τῃ βασιλικῃ, ὁν καλεισθαι Ζωγανην.

round the house, clothed in a royal garment, and him they call Zoganes. —*Athenæus*, lib. 14.

# MEGASTHENES:

## FROM ABYDENUS.

### OF NEBUCHADNEZZAR.

ΑΒΥΔΗΝΟΣ εν τη Ασσυριων γραφη, Μεγασθενης δε φησι. Ναβουκοδροσορον Ἡρακλεος αλκιμωτερον γεγονοτα επι τε Λιβυην και Ιβηριην στρατευσαι· ταυτας δε χειρωσαμενον αποδασμον αυτεων εις τα δεξια του ποντου κατοικισαι. Μετα δε λεγεται προς Χαλδαιων, ὡς αναβας επι τα βασιληΐα κατασχεθειη θεῳ ὁτεῳ δη. φθεγξαμενος δε ειπεν οὑτως. "Εγω Ναβουκοδροσορος, ω Βαβυλωνιοι, την μελλουσαν ὑμιν προαγγελλω συμφορην, την ουτε Βηλος εμος προγονος, ουτε βασιλεια Βηλτις αποτρεψαι μοιρας πεισαι σθενουσι. ἡξει Περσης ἡμιονος τοισι ὑμετεροισι δαιμοσι χρεωμενος συμμαχοισιν· επαξει δε δουλοσυνην. οὑ δη συναιτιος εσται Μηδης το Ασσυριον αυχημα. ὡς ειθε μιν προσθεν, η δουναι τους πολιητας, χαρυβδιν τινα η θαλασ-

Abydenus, in his history of the Assyrians, has preserved the following fragment of Megasthenes, who says: That Nabucodrosorus, having become more powerful than Hercules, invaded Libya and Iberia, and when he had rendered them tributary, he extended his conquests over the inhabitants of the shores upon the right of the sea. It is moreover related by the Chaldæans, that as he went up into his palace he was possessed by some god; and he cried out and said: "Oh! Babylonians, I, Nabucodrosorus, foretel unto you a calamity which must shortly come to pass, which neither Belus my ancestor, nor his queen Beltis, have power to persuade the Fates to turn away. A Persian mule shall come, and by the assistance of your gods shall impose upon you the yoke of slavery: the author of which shall be a Mede, the foolish pride of Assyria. Before he should thus betray my subσαν εισδεξαμενη αϊστωσαι προῤῥιζον, η μιν αλλας οδους στραφεντα φερεσθαι δια της ερημου, ινα ουτε αστεα, ουτε πατος ανθρωπων, θηρες δε νομον εχουσι, και ορνιθες πλαζονται, εν τε πετρῃσι και χαραδρῃσι μουνον αλωμενον· εμε τε πριν ες νοον βαλεσθαι ταυτα, τελεος αμεινονος κυρησαι."

Ὁ μεν θεσπισας παραχρημα ηφανιστο. ὁ δε οἱ παις Ευιλμαλουρουχος εβασιλευε. τον δε ὁ κηδεστης αποκτεινας Νηριγλισαρης λειπε παιδα, Λαβασσοαρασκον. τουτου δε αποθανοντος βιαιῳ μορῳ, Ναβαννιδοχον αποδεικνυσι βασιλεα, προσηκοντα οἱ ουδεν. τῳ δε Κυρος ἑλων Βαβυλωνα Καρμανιης ἡγεμονιην δωρεεται.

(Και περι του κτισαι δε τον Ναβουχοδονοσορ την Βαβυλωνα, ὁ αυτος ταυτα γραφει·) λεγεται δε παντα μεν εξ αρχης ὑδωρ ειναι, θαλασσαν καλεομενην. Βηλον δε σφεα παυσαι, χωρην ἑκαστῳ αποτειμαντα, και Βαβυλωνα τειχει περιβαλειν· τῳ χρονῳ δε τῳ ικνευμενῳ αφανισθηναι. τειχισαι δε αυθις Ναβουχοδονοσορον το μεχρι της Μακεδονων αρχης διαμειναν εον χαλκοπυλον. Και μεθ' ἑτερα επιλεγει, Να-

jects, Oh! that some sea or whirlpool might receive him, and his memory be blotted out for ever; or that he might be cast out to wander through some desert, where there are neither cities nor the trace of men, a solitary exile among rocks and caverns, where beasts and birds alone abide. But for me, before he shall have conceived these mischiefs in his mind, a happier end will be provided."

When he had thus prophesied, he expired: and was succeeded by his son Evilmaluruchus, who was slain by his kinsman Neriglisares: and Neriglisares left Labassoarascus his son: and when he also had suffered death by violence, they made Nabannidochus king, being no relation to the royal race: and in his reign Cyrus took Babylon, and granted him a principality in Carmania.

And concerning the rebuilding of Babylon by Nabuchodonosor, he writes thus: It is said that from the beginning all things were water, called the sea (Thalatth?): that Belus caused this state of things to cease, and appointed to each its proper place: and he surrounded Babylon with a wall: but in process of time this wall disappeared: and Nabuchodonosor walled it in again, and it remained so with its brazen gates until the time of the Macedonian conquest. And after other things he says: Naβουχοδονοσορος δε διαδεξαμενος την αρχην, Βαβυλωνα μεν ετειχισε τριπλῳ περιβολῳ, εν πεντεκαιδεκα ἡμερῃσι, τον δε Αρμακαλην ποταμον εξηγαγεν, εοντα κερας Ευφρητεω, τον τε Ακρακανον. ὑπερ δε της Σιππαρηνων πολιος, λακκον ορυξαμενος, περιμετρον μεν τεσσαρακοντα παρασαγγεων, βαθος δ' οργυιων εικοσι, πυλας επεστησεν, τας ανοιγοντες αρδεσκον το πεδιον· καλεουσι δ' αυτας εχετογνωμονας· επετειχισε δε και της Ερυθρης θαλασσης την επικλυσιν, και Τερηδονα πολιν εκτισεν, κατα τας Αραβων εισβολας· τα τε βασιληια δενδροις ησκησε, κρημαστους παραδεισους ονομασας.

buchodonosor having succeeded to the kingdom, built the walls of Babylon in a triple circuit in fifteen days; and he turned the river Armacale, a branch of the Euphrates, and the Acracanus: and above the city of Sippara he dug a receptacle for the waters, whose perimeter was forty parasangs, and whose depth was twenty cubits; and he placed gates at the entrance thereof, by opening which they irrigated the plains, and these they call Echetognomones (sluices:) and he constructed dykes against the irruptions of the Erythræan sea, and built the city of Teredon against the incursions of the Arabs; and he adorned the palace with trees, calling them hanging gardens.—*Euseb. Præp. Evan.* lib. 10.—*Euseb. Chron.* 19.

# THE FRAGMENTS

OF

# THE EGYPTIAN HISTORIES:

CONTAINING

THE HERMETIC CREED;
THE OLD CHRONICLE;
THE REMAINS OF MANETHO;
AND
THE LATERCULUS OF ERATOSTHENES.

# THE HERMETIC CREED:

ΠΡΟ των οντως οντων, και των ὁλων αρχων, εϛι θεος εἱς, πρωτος και του πρωτου Θεου και βασιλεως, ακινητος εν μονοτητι της ἑαυτου ενοτητος μενων, ουτε γαρ νοητον αυτῳ επιπλεκεται, ουτε αλλο τι. Παραδειγμα δε ἱδρυται του αυτου πατρος, αυτογονου, και μονοπατορος Θεου, του οντως αγαθου. Μειζον γαρ τε και πρωτον, και πηγη των παντων, και πυθμην των νοουμενων πρωτων ειδων οντων. Απο δε του ἑνος τουτου, ὁ αυταρχης Θεος ἑαυτον εξελαμψε· διο και αυτοπατωρ και αυταρχης. Αρχη γαρ αυτος και Θεος Θεων. Μονας εκ του ἑνος, προ ουσιας, και Αρχη της ουσιας· απ' αυτου γαρ ἡ ουσιοτης και ἡ ουσια· διο και νοηταρχης προσαγορευεται. Αυται μεν ουν εισιν αρχαι πρεσβυταται

BEFORE all things that really exist, and before the beginning of all time, there is one God, prior to the first God, and ruler of the world, remaining immoveable in the solitude of his unity; for neither is intelligence immixed with him, nor any other thing. He is the exemplar of himself; the Father, the self-begotten God, who is the only Father, and is truly good. For he is the greatest and the first, the fountain of all things and the root of all primary intellectual forms. But out of this one, the God that is self-sufficient shone forth of himself: for which reason he is the father of himself, and all-sufficient: for he is the beginning and the God of gods. He is unity from the only one; before essence, and yet he is the beginning of essence, for from him is entity and essence; on which account he is celebrated as the prince of intelliπαντων, ὡς Ἑρμης προ των αιθεριων και εμπυριων Θεων προταττει και των επουρανιων.

gence. These are the most ancient principles of all things, which Hermes places first in order, before the ethereal, empyrean, and celestial deities. —*Jamblichus.*

# THE OLD EGYPTIAN CHRONICLE:

ΦΕΡΕΤΑΙ γαρ Αιγυπτιοις παλαιον τι χρονογραφειον περιεχον λ′. δυναστειων εν γενεαις παλιν ριγ′. χρονων απειρων, εν μυριασι, τρισι, και ,εφκε′. πρωτον μεν των Αυριτων, δευτερον δε των Μεστραιων, τριτον δε Αιγυπτιων· ούτω πως επι λεξεως εχον.

Ἡφαιστου χρονος ουκ εστιν· δια το νυκτος και ἡμερας αυτον φαινειν.

Ἡλιος Ἡφαιστου εβασιλευσεν ετων μυριαδας τρεις.

Επειτα Κρονος (φησι) και οἱ λοιποι παντες θεοι δωδεκα εβασιλευσεν ετη, ,γϡπδ′.

Επειτα ἡμιθεοι βασιλεις οκτω ετη σιζ′.

Και μετ' αυτους γενεαι ιε′. Κυνικου κυκλου ανεγραφησαν εν ετεσι υμγ′.

Ειτα Τανιτων ις′. δυναστεια, γενεων η′. ετων ρϙ′.

Among the Egyptians there is a certain tablet called the Old Chronicle, containing thirty dynasties in 113 descents, during the long period of 36525 years. The first series of princes was that of the Auritæ; the second was that of the Mestræans; the third of Egyptians. The Chronicle runs as follows:

To Hephæstus is assigned no time, as he is apparent both by night and day.

Helius the son of Hephæstus reigned three myriads of years.

Then Cronus and the other twelve divinities reigned 3984 years.

Next in order are the demigods, in number eight, who reigned 217 years.

After these are enumerated 15 generations of the Cynic circle, which take up 443 years.

The 16th Dynasty is of the Tanites, eight kings, which lasted 190 years.

| | |
|---|---|
| Προς οἱς ιζ΄. δυναςεια Μεμφιτων, γενεων δ΄. ετων ργ΄. | 17th Memphites, 4 in descent, 103 years. |
| Μεθ' οἱς ιη΄. δυναςεια Μεμφιτων, γενεων ιδ΄. ετων τμη΄. | 18th Memphites, 14 in descent, 348 years. |
| Επειτα ιθ΄ δυναστεια Διοσπολιτων, γενεων ε΄. ετων ρϟδ΄. | 19th Diospolites, 5 in descent, 194 years. |
| Ειτα εικοστη δυναστεια Διοσπολιτων, γενεων η΄. ετων σκη΄. | 20th Diospolites, 8 in descent, 228 years. |
| Επειτα κα΄. δυναστεια Ταvιτων, γενεων ϛ΄. ετων ρκα΄. | 21st Tanites, . 6 in descent, 121 years. |
| Ειτα κβ΄. δυναστεια Ταvιτων, γενεων γ΄. ετων μη΄. | 22nd Tanites, . 3 in descent, 48 years. |
| κγ΄. δυναστεια Διοσπολιτων, γενεων β΄. ετων ιθ΄. | 23rd Diospolites, 2 in descent, 19 years. |
| Ειτα κδ΄. δυναστεια Σαϊτων, γενεων γ΄. ετων μδ΄. | 24th Saïtes, . 3 in descent, 44 years. |
| Προς οἱς κε΄. δυναστεια Αιθιοπων, γενεων γ΄. ετων μδ΄. | 25th Ethiopians, 3 in descent, 44 years. |
| Μεθ' οἱς κϛ΄. δυναστεια Μεμφιτων, γενεων ζ΄. ετων ροζ΄. | 26th Memphites, 7 in descent, 177 years. |
| Και μετα τουτους κζ΄. Περσων ε΄. ετων ρκδ΄. | 27th Persians . 5 in descent, 124 years. |
| κη΄. | 28th |
| Επειτα κθ΄. δυναστεια Ταvιτων, γενεων, ετων λθ΄. | 29th Tanites, . in descent, 39 years. |
| Και επι πασαις λ΄. δυναστεια Ταvιτου ἑνος, ετων ιη΄. | 30th a Tanite, . 1 in descent, 18 years. |
| Τα παντα ὁμου των λ΄. δυναστειων ετη μυριαδας γ΄. και ϛφκε΄. | In all, 30 Dynasties, and 36525 years.—*Syncel. Chron.* 51.—***Euseb.*** *Chron.* 6. |

# MANETHO:

## THE EPISTLE OF MANETHO, THE SEBENNYTE, TO PTOLEMY PHILADELPHUS.

**ΒΑΣΙΛΕΙ** μεγαλῳ Πτολεμαιῳ Φιλαδελφῳ σεϐαστῳ, Μανεθω αρχιερευς και γραμματευς των κατ' Αιγυπτον ἱερων αδυτων, γενει Σεϐεννυτης ὑπαρχων, Ἡλιουπολιτης, τῳ δεσποτῃ μου Πτολεμαιῳ. Χαιρειν.

Ἡμας δει λογιζεσθαι, μεγιστε βασιλευ, περι παντων ὡν εαν βουλῃ ἡμας εξετασαι πραγματων· επιζητουντι σοι περι των μελλοντων τῳ κοσμῳ γιγνεσθαι καθετος καλευσας μοι περιφανησεται σοι ἁ εμαθον ἱερα βιϐλια γραφεντα ὑπο των προπατορος τρισμεγιστου Ἑρμου, Ερρωσο μοι, Δεσποτα μου Βασιλευ.

To the great and august king Ptolemy Philadelphus: Manetho, the high priest and scribe of the sacred adyta in Egypt, being by birth a Sebennyte and a citizen of Heliopolis, to his sovereign Ptolemy, humbly greeting:

It is right for us, most mighty king, to pay due attention to all things which it is your pleasure we should take into consideration. In answer then to your inquiries concerning the things which shall come to pass in the world, I shall, according to your commands, lay before you what I have gathered from the sacred books written by Hermes Trismegistus, our forefather. Farewell, my prince and sovereign. — *Syncel. Chron.* 40.— *Euseb. Chron.* 6.

# THE EGYPTIAN DYNASTIES.

## THE DYNASTY OF THE DEMIGODS.

| | |
|---|---|
| Αιγυπτιων α'. εϐασιλευσεν Ἡφαιστος ετη ψκδ'. ἡμισυ και τεσσαρας ἡμερας. | The 1st of the Egyptian kings was Hephæstus, who reigned 724 years and a half and 4 days. |
| Αιγυπτιων β'. εϐασιλευσεν Ἡλιος Ἡφαιστου ετη πϛ' | The 2nd was Helius, the son of Hephæstus, 86 years. |
| Αιγυπτιων γ'. εϐασιλευσεν Αγαθοδαιμων ετη νϛ'. και ἡμισυ και δεκα ἡμερας. | 3rd, Agathodæmon, who reigned 56 and a half and ten days. |
| Αιγυπτιων δ'. εϐασιλευσεν Κρονος ετη μ'. και ἡμισυ. | 4th, Cronus, 40 and a half years. |
| Αιγυπτιων ε'. εϐασιλευσεν Οσιρις και Ισις ετη λε'. | 5th, Osiris and Isis, 35 years. |
| Αιγυπτιων ϛ'. εϐασιλευσεν ετη. | 6th, . . . years. |
| Αιγυπτιων ζ'. εϐασιλευσεν Τυφων ετη κθ'. | 7th, Typhon, 29 years. |
| Αιγυπτιων η'. εϐασιλευσεν Ὡρος ἡμιθεος ετη κε'. | 8th, Horus, the demigod, 25 years. |
| Αιγυπτιων θ'. εϐασιλευσεν Αρης ἡμιθεος ετη κγ'. | 9th, Ares, the demigod, 23 years. |
| Αιγυπτιων ι'. εϐασιλευσεν Ανουϐις ἡμιθεος ετη ιζ'. | 10th, Anubis, the demigod, 17 years. |
| Αιγυπτιων ια'. εϐασιλευσεν Ἡρακλης ἡμιθεος ετη ιε'. | 11th, Heracles, the demigod, 15 years. |
| Αιγυπτιων ιϐ'. εϐασιλευσεν Απολλω ἡμιθεος ετη κε' | 12th, Apollo, the demigod, 25 years. |

Αιγυπτιων ιγ'. εβασιλευσεν Αμμων ἡμιθεος ετη λ'.

13th, Ammon, the demigod, 30 years.

Αιγυπτιων ιδ'. εβασιλευσεν Τιθοης ἡμιθεος ετη κζ'.

14th, Tithoes, the demigod, 27 years.

Αιγυπτιων ιε'. εβασιλευσεν Σωσος ἡμιθεος ετη λβ'.

15th, Sosus, the demigod, 32 years.

Αιγυπτιων ις'. εβασιλευσεν Ζευς ἡμιθεος ετη κ'.

16th, Zeus, the demigod, 20 years.—*Syncel. Chron.* 19.—*Euseb. Chron.* 7.

## THE EGYPTIAN DYNASTIES AFTER THE DELUGE.

### THE FIRST DYNASTY.

α'. Μετα νεκυας τους ἡμιθεους πρωτη βασιλεια καταριθμειται βασιλεων οκτω, ὡν πρωτος Μηνης Θεεινιτης εβασιλευσεν ετη ξβ'. ὁς ὑπο Ἱπποποταμου διαπραγεις διεφθαρη.

1. After the dead demigods the first dynasty consisted of eight kings, of whom the first was Menes the Thinite; he reigned 62 years, and perished by a wound received from an hippopotamus.

β'. Αθωθις (Αθωσθις)* υἱος ετη νζ'. ὁ τα εν Μεμφει βασιλεια οικοδομησας· οὑ φερονται βιβλοι ανατομικαι, ιατρος γαρ ην.

2. Athothis, his son, reigned 57 years; he built the palaces at Memphis, and left the anatomical books, for he was a physician.

γ'. Κενκενης (Κερκενης) υἱος ετη λα'.

3. Cencenes, his son, reigned 31 years.

δ'. Ουενεφης (Ουενεφρης) υἱος ετη κγ'. εφ'. οὑ λιμος κατεσχεν την Αιγυπτον μεγας. οὑτος παρα Κωχωμην ηγειρε πυραμιδας.

4. Venephes, his son, reigned 23 years. In his time a great plague raged through Egypt. He raised the pyramids near Cochome.

ε'. Ουσαφαιδος (Ουσαφαης) υἱος ετη κ'.

5. Usaphædus, his son, reigned 20 years.

* The names and paragraphs contained between the parentheses are the variations which occur in Eusebius.

| | |
|---|---|
| ϛ'. Μιεβιδος (Νιεβης) υἱος ετη κϛ'. | 6. Miebidus, his son, 26 years. |
| ζ'. Σεμεμψις (Σεμεμψης) υἱος ετη ιη'. εφ' οὑ φθορα μεγιστη κατεσχεν την Αιγυπτον. | 7. Semempsis, his son, reigned 18 years. In his reign a terrible pestilence afflicted Egypt. |
| η'. Βιηναχης (Ουβιεντης) υἱος ετη κϛ'. | 8. Bienaches, his son reigned 26 years. |
| Ομου ετη σνγ'. | The whole number of years amounted to 253. |

## THE SECOND DYNASTY.

| | |
|---|---|
| Δευτερα δυναστεια Θεινιτων βασιλεων εννεα ὡν. | Of nine Thinite kings. |
| α'. Πρωτος Βοηθος (Βωχος) ετη λη'. εφ' οὑ χασμα κατα Βουβαστον εγενετο, και απωλοντο πολλοι. | 1. Boethus the first reigned 38 years. During his reign a chasm of the earth opened near Bubastus, and many persons perished. |
| β'. Καιαχως (Χοος) ετη λθ'. εφ' οὑ οἱ βοες Απις εν Μεμφει, και Μνευις εν Ἡλιουπολει, και ὁ Μενδησιος τραγος ενομισθησαν ειναι θεοι. | 2. Cæachos reigned 39 years. Under him the bulls Apis in Memphis, and Meneus in Heliopolis, and the Mendesian goat, were appointed to be gods. |
| γ'. Βινωθρις (Βιοφις) ετη μζ'. εφ' οὑ εκριθη τας γυναικας βασιλειας γερας εχειν. | 3. Binothris reigned 47 years. In whose time it was judged that women might hold the imperial government. |
| δ'. Τλας ετη ιζ'. | 4. Tlas reigned 17 years. |
| ε'. Σεθενης ετη μα'. | 5. Sethenes reigned 41 years. |
| ϛ'. Χαιρης ετη ιζ'. | 6. Chæres 17 years. |
| ζ'. Νεφερχερης ετη κε'. εφ' οὑ μυθευεται τον Νειλον μελιτι κεκραμμενον ἡμερας ἑνδεκα ῥυηναι. | 7. Nephercheres 25 years. In his time it is said the Nile flowed with honey during eleven days. |
| (η'. Σεσωχρις ετη μη', ὁς ὑψος ειχε πηχων ε'. πλατος γ'. | (8. Sesochris 48 years, whose height was five cubits, and his breadth three. |

θ'. Χενερης ετη λ'.
(Ομου ετη τϐ'.)

9. Chencres 30 years.
The whole number of years is 302.)

## THE THIRD DYNASTY.

Τριτη δυναστεια Μεμφιτων βασιλεων εννεα· ὡν

α'. Νεχεροφης (Νεχερωχις) ετη κη'. εφ' οὗ Λιβυες απεστησαν Αιγυπτιων, και της σεληνης παρα λογον αυξηθεισης, δια δεος ἑαυτους παρεδοσαν.

β'. Τοσορθρος (Σεσορθος) ετη κθ'. οὗτος Ασκληπιος Αιγυπτιοις κατα την ιατρικην νενομισται, και την δια ξεστων λιθων οικοδομιαν εὗρατο, αλλα και γραφης επεμεληθη.

γ'. Τυρις ετη ζ'.
δ'. Μεσωχρις ετη ιζ'.
ε'. Σωϊφις ετη ις'.
ϛ'. Τοσερτασις ετη ιθ'.
ζ'. Αχις ετη μϐ'.
η'. Σιφουρις ετη λ'.
θ'. Κερφερης ετη κϛ'.
Ομου εστιν σιδ'.

Of nine Memphite kings.

1. Necherophes reigned 28 years. In his time the Libyans revolted from the Egyptians, but on account of an unexpected increase of the moon they surrendered themselves for fear.

2. Tosorthrus reigned 29 years. He is called Asclepius by the Egyptians, for his medical knowledge. He built a house of hewn stones, and greatly patronized writing.

3. Tyris reigned 7 years.
4. Mesochris 17 years.
5. Soïphis 16 years.
6. Tosertasis 19 years.
7. Achis 42 years.
8. Siphuris 30 years.
9. Cerpheres 26 years.
Altogether 214 years.

## THE FOURTH DYNASTY.

Τεταρτη δυναστεια Μεμφιτων συγγενειας ἑτερας βασιλεις η'.

α'. Σωρις ετη κθ'.
β'. Σουφις ετη ξγ'. ὁς την

Of eight Memphite kings of a different race.

1. Soris reigned 29 years.
2. Suphis reigned 63 years. He

μεγιστην ηγειρε πυραμιδα, ούτος δε και ὁ Περοπτης εις θεους εγενετο και την ἱεραν συνεγραφε βιβλον.

γ'. Σουφις ετη ξϛ'.
δ'. Μενχερης ετη ξγ'.
ε'. Ρατοισης ετη κε'.
ϛ'. Βιχερης ετη κβ'.
ζ'. Σεβερχερης ετη ζ'.
η'. Θαμφθις ετη θ'.
Ὁμου ετη σοδ'.

built the largest pyramid: he was called also Peroptes, and was translated to the gods, and wrote the sacred book.

3. Suphis reigned 66 years
4. Mencheres 63 years.
5. Ratœses 25 years.
6. Bicheres 22 years.
7. Sebercheres 7 years.
8. Thampthis 9 years.
Altogether 274 years.

## THE FIFTH DYNASTY.

Πεμπτη δυναστεια βασιλεων εξ Ελεφαντινης.

α'. Ουσερχερις ετη κη'.
β'. Σεφρης ετη ιγ'.
γ'. Νεφερχερης ετη κ'.
δ'. Σισιρις ετη ζ'.
ε'. Χερης ετη κ'.
ϛ'. Ραθουρις ετη μδ'.
ζ'. Μερχερης ετη θ'.
η'. Ταρχερης ετη μδ'.
θ'. Οβνος ετη λγ'.
Ὁμου ετη σμη'.

Of nine Elephantine kings.

1. Usercheris reigned 28 years.
2. Sephres 13 years.
3. Nephercheres 20 years.
4. Sisiris 7 years.
5. Cheres 20 years.
6. Rathuris 44 years.
7. Mercheres 9 years.
8. Tarcheres 44 years.
9. Obnos 33 years.
Altogether 248 years.

## THE SIXTH DYNASTY.

Ἑκτη δυναστεια βασιλεων ἐξ Μεμφιτων.

α'. Οθωης, (Θωης) ὁς ὑπο δορυφορων αναιρεθη.
β'. Φιος ετη νγ'.

Of six Memphite kings.

1. Othoes, who was killed by his guards.
2. Phius reigned 53 years.

γ'. Μεθουσουφις ετη ζ'.

3. Methusuphis 7 years.

δ'. Φιωψ (Αφιωψ) ἑξαετης αρξαμενος βασιλευειν. διεγενετο μεχρις ετων ρ'.

4. Phiops who began to reign at six years of age, and reigned till he had completed his hundredth year.

ε'. Μεντεσουφις ετος ἑν.

5. Mentesuphis reigned one year.

ϛ'. Νιτωκρις γεννικωτατη, και ευμορφοτατη των κατ' αυτην γενομενη, ξανθη την χροιαν ἡ την τριτην ηγειρε πυραμιδα· εβασιλευσεν ετη ιβ'.

6. Nitocris, who was the most handsome woman of her time, of a dark complexion; she built the third pyramid, and reigned 12 years.

Ομου ετη σγ'.

Altogether 203 years.

## THE SEVENTH DYNASTY.

Ἑβδομη δυναστεια Μεμφιτων βασιλεων ο'. οἱ εβασιλευσαν ἡμερας ο'.

Of seventy Memphite kings, who reigned 70 days.

## THE EIGHTH DYNASTY.

Ογδοη δυναστεια Μεμφιτων βασιλεων κζ'. οἱ εβασιλευσαν ετη ρμϛ'.

Of twenty-seven Memphite kings, who reigned 146 years.

## THE NINTH DYNASTY.

Εννατη δυναστεια Ἡρακλεωτικων βασιλεων ιθ'. οἱ εβασιλευσαν ετη υθ'. ὡν

Of nineteen Heracleotic kings, who reigned 409 years.

Ὁ πρωτος Αχθοης δεινοτατος των προ αυτου γενομενος, τοις εν παση Αιγυπτῳ κακα ειργασατο, μανιᾳ περιεπεσεν, και ὑπο κροκοδειλου διεφθαρη.

1. The first was Achthoes, the worst of all his predecessors. He did much harm to all the inhabitants of Egypt, was seized with madness, and killed by a crocodile.

## THE TENTH DYNASTY.

Δεκατη δυναστεια Ἡρακλεωτικων βασιλεων ιθʹ. οἱ εβασιλευσαν ρπεʹ.

Of 19 Heracleotic kings, who reigned 185 years.

## THE ELEVENTH DYNASTY.

Ἑνδεκατη δυναστεια Διοσπολιτων βασιλεων ιϛʹ. οἱ εβασιλευσαν ετη μγʹ. μεθ' οἷς Αμμενεμης ετη ιϛʹ.

Ὁμου βασιλεις, ρϟβʹ. ετη, ͵βτηʹ. ἡμερας οʹ.

Of sixteen Diospolites kings, who reigned 43 years. Among whom Ammenemes reigned 16 years.

The whole number of the abovementioned kings is 192, who reigned during a space of 2308 years and 70 days. — *Syncel. Chron.* 54 to 59. —*Euseb. Chron.* 14, 15.

# THE SECOND BOOK OF MANETHO:

## THE TWELFTH DYNASTY.

ΔΩΔΕΚΑΤΗ δυναστεια Διοσπολιτων βασιλεων ἑπτα.

α΄. Γεσων Γωσης Αμμανεμου (Σεσογχωρις Αμμενεμου) υἱος· ετη μϛ΄.

β΄. Αμμανεμης (Αμμενεμης) ετη λη΄. ὁς ὑπο των ιδιων ευνουχων ανηρεθη.

γ΄. Σεσωστρις ετη μη΄. ὁς ἁπασαν εχειρωσατο την Ασιαν εν ενιαυτοις εννεα, και της Ευρωπης τα μεχρι Θρακης πανταχοσε μνημοσυνα εγειρας της των εθνων κατασχεσεως· επι μεν τοις γενναιοις, ανδρων· επι δε τοις αγεννεσι, γυναικων μορια ταις στηλαις εγχαραττων, ὡς ὑπο Αιγυπτιων μετα Οσιριν πρωτον νομισθηναι.

δ΄. Λαχαρης (Λαβαρις) ετη η΄. ὁς τον εν Αρσενοΐτῃ λαβυρινθον ἑαυτῳ ταφον κατεσκευασεν.

Of seven Diospolite kings.

1. Geson Goses the son of Ammanemes. He reigned 46 years.

2. Ammanemes reigned 38 years. He was slain by his eunuchs.

3. Sesostris 48 years. He conquered all Asia in nine years, and Europe as far as Thrace, every where erecting monuments of his conquests of those nations; of men among nations who acted bravely, but among the degenerate he erected figures of women, engraving their follies upon the pillars. By the Egyptians he is supposed to be the first after Osiris.

4. Lachares 8 years, who built the Labyrinth in Arsenoïte as a tomb for himself.

| | |
|---|---|
| ε'. Αμμερης ετη η'. | 5. Ammeres 8 years. |
| ϛ'. Αμμενεμης ετη η'. | 6. Ammenemes 8 years. |
| ζ'. Σκεμιοφρις αδελφη ετη δ'. | 7. Scemiophris, his sister, 4 years. |
| Ομου ετη ρξ'. | Altogether 160 years. |

## THE THIRTEENTH DYNASTY.

| | |
|---|---|
| Τρισκαιδεκατη δυναστεια Διοσπολιτων βασιλεων ξ'. οἱ εβασιλευσαν ρπδ'. ετη. | Of 60 Diospolite kings, who reigned 184 years. |
| Λειπει. | The names are lost. |

## THE FOURTEENTH DYNASTY.

Is lost altogether.

## THE FIFTEENTH DYNASTY.

| | |
|---|---|
| Πεντεδεκατη* ποιμενων. | Of the Shepherds. |
| Ησαν δε Φοινικες ξενοι βασιλεις ϛ'. οἱ και Μεμφιν εἱλον. οἱ και εν τῳ Σεθροΐτῃ νομῳ πολιν εκτισαν, αφ' ἡς ὁρμωμενοι Αιγυπτιους εχειρωσαντο, ὧν | There were six foreign Phœnician kings: they took Memphis, and built a city in the Sethroïte nome, from whence they made an invasion, and conquered all Egypt; of whom |
| α'. Σαΐτης εβασιλευσεν ετη ιθ'. αφ' οὑ και ὁ Σαΐτης νομος. | 1. Saïtes reigned 19 years, after whom the Saïte Nome is so called. |
| β'. Βεων (Βνων Ανων) ετη μδ'. | 2. Beon reigned 44 years. |
| γ'. Παχναν (Αφωφις) ετη ξα'. | 3. Pachnan 61 years. |
| δ'. Σταν ετη ν'. | 4. Staan 50 years. |
| ε'. Αρχλης (Ανχλης) ετη μθ'. | 5. Archles 49 years. |

* This is the seventeenth according to Eusebius.

| | |
|---|---|
| ϛʹ. Αφοβις ετη ξαʹ. | 6. Aphobis 61 years. |
| Ομου ετη σπδʹ. | Altogether 284 years. |

## THE SIXTEENTH DYNASTY.

| | |
|---|---|
| 'Εκκαιδεκατη δυναστεια ποιμενες 'Ελληνες βασιλεις λβʹ. εβασιλευσαν ετη φιηʹ. | Of 32 Grecian shepherds, who reigned 518 years. |

## THE SEVENTEENTH DYNASTY.

| | |
|---|---|
| 'Επτακαιδεκατη δυναστεια ποιμενες αλλοι βασιλεις μγʹ. Και Θηβαιοι Διοσπολιται μγʹ. | Consisted of 43 shepherd kings and 43 Theban Diospolites. |
| Ομου οἱ ποιμενες, και οἱ Θηβαιοι εβασιλευσαν ετη ρναʹ. | The Shepherds and Thebans reigned altogether 151 years. |

## THE EIGHTEENTH DYNASTY.

| | |
|---|---|
| Οκτωκαιδεκατη δυναστεια Διοσπολιτων βασιλεων ιϛʹ. ὧν | Of sixteen Diospolite kings. |
| αʹ. Πρωτος Αμως (Αμωσις ετη κεʹ.) | 1. Amos. |
| βʹ. Χεβρως (Χεβρων) ετη ιγʹ. | 2. Chebros 13 years. |
| γʹ. Αμενωφθις (Αμμενωφις) ετη κδʹ. | 3. Amenophthis 24 years. |
| δʹ. Αμερσις (Μιφρις) ετη κβʹ. | 4. Amersis 22 years. |
| εʹ. Μισαφρις* ετη ιγʹ. | 5. Misaphris 13 years. |
| ϛʹ. Μισφραγμουθωσις ετη | 6. Misphragmathosis 26 years, in |

* In the list of Eusebius the fifth is omitted, and the name of Χεβρης inserted between the thirteenth and fourteenth.

| | |
|---|---|
| κϛʹ. εφʹ ού ὁ επι Δευκαλιωνος κατακλυσμος. | whose time happened the deluge of Deucalion. |
| ζʹ. Τουθμωσις ετη θʹ. | 7. Tuthmosis 9 years. |
| ηʹ. Αμενωφις ετη λαʹ. οὗτος εστιν ὁ Μεμνων ειναι νομιζομενος, και φθεγγομενος λιθος. | 8. Amenophis 31 years. He is supposed to be Memnon, to whom the musical statue is erected. |
| θʹ. Ὡρος ετη λζʹ. | 9. Horus 37 years. |
| ιʹ. Αχεῤῥης (Αχενχερσης) ετη λϐʹ. | 10. Acherrhes 32 years. |
| ιαʹ. Ραθως (Αθωρις) ετη ἑξʹ. | 11. Rathos 6 years. |
| ιϐʹ. Χεϐρης (Χενχερης) ετη ιϐʹ. | 12. Chebres 12 years. |
| ιγʹ. Αχεῤῥης (Αχεῤῥης) ετη ιϐʹ. | 13. Acherrhes 12 years. |
| ιδʹ. Αρμεσης (Αρμαϊς ὁ Δαναος) ετη εʹ. | 14. Armeses 5 years. |
| ιεʹ. Ραμμεσσης (Αμμεσης ὁ και Αιγυπτος) ετος ἑν. | 15. Rammesses 1 year. |
| ιϛʹ. Αμενωφ (Μενωφις) ετη ιθʹ. | 16. Amenoph 19 years. |
| Ομου ετη σξγʹ. | Altogether 263 years. |

## THE NINETEENTH DYNASTY.

| | |
|---|---|
| Εννεακαιδεκατη δυναστεια βασιλεων ζʹ. Διοσπολιτων. | Of seven Diospolite kings. |
| αʹ. Σεθως ετη ναʹ. | 1. Sethos reigned 51 years. |
| βʹ. Ραψακης (ραψης) ετη ξαʹ. | 2. Rapsaces 61 years. |
| γʹ. Αμμενεφθης (Αμενωφθις) ετη κʹ. | 3. Ammenephthes 20 years. |
| δʹ. Ραμεσης ετη ξʹ. | 4. Rameses 60 years. |
| εʹ. Αμμενεμνης (Αμμενεμνης) ετη εʹ. | 5. Ammenemnes 5 years. |
| ϛʹ. Θουωρις, ὁ παρʹ Ὁμηρῳ καλουμενος Πολυϐους ϛʹ. | 6. Thuoris, who is called by Homer Polybus. |

ζ'. Αλκανδρος εφ' οὗ το Ιλιον ἑαλω ετη ζ'.

Ομου ετη σθ'.

Επι του αυτου δευτερου τομου, βασιλεις ϟϛ'. ετη ͵βρκα'.

7. Alcandrus 7 years, in whose time Ilion was taken.

Altogether 209 years.

In this second book of Manetho are contained 96 kings and 2121 years.—*Syncel. Chron.* 59 *to* 75.—*Euseb. Chron.* 15 *to* 17.

# THE THIRD BOOK OF MANETHO:

## THE TWENTIETH DYNASTY.

| | |
|---|---|
| ΕΙΚΟΣΤΗ δυναστεια βασιλεων Διοσπολιτων ιβ'. οἱ ἐβασιλευσαν ετη ρλε'. | Of 12 Diospolite kings, who reigned 135 years. |

## THE TWENTY-FIRST DYNASTY.

| | |
|---|---|
| Πρωτη και εικοστη δυναστεια βασιλεων Τανιτων ζ'. | Of seven Tanite kings. |
| α'. Σμεδης (Σμενδης) ετη κς'. | 1. Smedes reigned 26 years. |
| β'. Ψουσενης, η Ψουνεσης (Ψουσεννης) ετη μς'. | 2. Psusenes, or Psuneses, 46 years. |
| γ'. Νεφελχερης (Νεφερχερης) ετη δ'. | 3. Nephelcheres 4 years. |
| δ'. Αμενενωφθις (Αμενωφθις) ετη θ'. | 4. Amenophthis 9 years. |
| ε'. Οσοχορ (Οσοχωρ) ετη ς'. | 5. Osochor 6 years. |
| ς'. Πιναχης (Ψιναχης) ετη θ'. | 6. Pinaches 9 years. |
| ζ'. Σουσεννης (Ψουσεννης) ετη λ'. | 7. Susenes 30 years. |
| Ομου ετη ρλ'. | Altogether 130 years. |

## THE TWENTY-SECOND DYNASTY.

| | |
|---|---|
| Εικοστη δευτερα δυναστεια Βουβαστιτων βασιλεων θ'. | Of nine Bubastite kings. |
| Πρωτος Σεσογχις (Σεσεγχωσις) ετη κα'. | 1. Sesonchis 21 years. |
| β'. Οσωρωθ (Οσορθων) ετη ιε'. | 2. Osoroth 15 years. |
| γ'. δ'. ε'. Αλλοι τρεις ετη κε'. | 3, 4, 5. Three others reigned 25 years. |
| ς'. Τακελλωθις ετη ιγ'. | 6. Tacellothis 13 years. |
| ζ'. η'. θ'. Αλλοι τρεις ετη μβ'. | 7, 8, 9. Three others 42 years. |
| Ομου ετη ρκ'. | Altogether reigned 120 years. |

## THE TWENTY-THIRD DYNASTY.

| | |
|---|---|
| ΚΓ'. δυναστεια Τανιτων βασιλεων δ'. | Of four Tanite kings. |
| α'. Πετουβατης (Πετουβαστης) ετη μ'. εφ' ου Ολυμπιας ηχθη πρωτη. | 1. Petoubates reigned 40 years, in whose time the Olympiads began. |
| β'. Οσορχω (Οσορθων) ετη η'. δν 'Ηρακλεα Αιγυπτιοι καλουσιν. | 2. Osorcho 8 years, whom the Egyptians call Hercules. |
| γ'. Ψαμμους ετη ι'. | 3. Psammus 10 years. |
| δ'. Ζητ ετη λα'. | 4. Zeet 31 years. |
| Ομου ετη πθ'. | Altogether 89 years. |

## THE TWENTY-FOURTH DYNASTY.

| | |
|---|---|
| ΚΔ'. δυναστεια. | |
| Βοχχωρις (Βοκχωρις) Σαιτης | Bonchoris the Saite reigned 6 |

| | |
|---|---|
| ετη ϛ'. εφ' οὑ αρνιον εφθεγξατο ετη ϡϞ'. | years, in whose reign a sheep spoke. 990 years. |

## THE TWENTY-FIFTH DYNASTY.

| | |
|---|---|
| ΚΕ'. δυναστεια Αιθιοπων βασιλεων τριων. | Of three Ethiop kings. |
| α'. Σαββακων, ὁς αιχμαλωτον Βοχχωριν ἑλων εκαυσε ζωντα, και εβασιλευσεν ετη η'. | 1. Sabbacon, who having taken Bonchoris a captive, burnt him alive, and reigned 8 years. |
| β'. Σευηχος υἱος ετη ιδ'. | 2. Seuechus, his son, reigned 14 years. |
| γ'. Ταρκος (Ταρακος) ετη ιη'. | 3. Tarcus 18 years. |
| Ομου ετη μ'. | Altogether 40 years. |

## THE TWENTY-SIXTH DYNASTY.

| | |
|---|---|
| Ἑκτη και εικοστη δυναστεια Σαϊτων βασιλεων εννεα. | Of nine Saite kings. |
| α'. Στεφινατης (Στεφαναθις) ετη ζ'. | 1. Stephinates reigned 7 years. |
| β'. Νερεψος (Νεχεψος) ετη ϛ'. | 2. Nerepsos 6 years. |
| γ'. Νεχαω ετη η'. | 3. Nechao 8 years. |
| δ'. Ψαμμιτικος (Ψαμμιτιχος) ετη νδ'. | 4. Psammiticus 54 years. |
| ε'. Νεχαω δευτερος ετη ϛ'. οὑτος εἱλε την Ἱερουσαλημ, και Ιωαχαζ τον βασιλεα εις Αιγυπτον απηγαγεν. | 5. Nechao the second 6 years. He took Jerusalem, and carried Joachas, the king, to Egypt. |
| ϛ'. Ψαμμουθις ἑτερος ετη ιζ'. | 6. Psammuthius 6 years. |
| ζ'. Ουαφρις (Ουαφρης) ετη ιθ'. ᾧ προσεφυγον ἁλουσης ὑπο | 7. Vaphris 19 years, to whom the remainder of the Jews fled when |

| | |
|---|---|
| Ασσυριων Ἱερουσαλημ οἱ των Ιουδαιων ὑπολοιποι. | Jerusalem was taken by the Assyrians. |
| η΄. Αμωσις ετη μδ΄. | 8. Amosis 44 years. |
| θ΄. Ψαμμαχεριτης* μηνας ς΄. | 9. Psammacherites 6 months. |
| Ομου ετη ρν΄. και μηνας ς΄. | Altogether 150 years and six months. |

## THE TWENTY-SEVENTH DYNASTY.

| | |
|---|---|
| ΚΖ΄. βασιλεια Περσων βασιλεων η΄. | Of eight Persian kings. |
| α΄. Καμβυσης ετη ε΄. της ἑαυτου βασιλειας. Περσων εβασιλευσεν Αιγυπτου ετη ς΄. | 1. Cambyses reigned over Persia, his own kingdom, 5 years, and over Egypt 6 years. |
| β΄. Δαρειος Ὑστασπου ετη λς΄. | 2. Darius, the son of Hystaspes, 36 years. |
| γ. Ξερξης ὁ μεγας ετη κα΄. | 3. Xerxes the Great 21 years. |
| δ΄. Αρταβανος† μηνας ζ΄. | 4. Artabanus 7 months. |
| ε΄. Αρταξερξης ετη μα΄. | 5. Artaxerxes 41 years. |
| ς΄. Ξερξης μηνας δυο. | 6. Xerxes 2 months. |
| ζ΄. Σογδιανος μηνας ζ΄. | 7. Sogdianus 7 months. |
| η΄. Δαρειος Ξερξου ιθ΄. | 8. Darius the son of Xerxes, 19 years. |
| Ομου ετη ρκδ΄. μηνας δ΄. | Altogether 124 years and four months. |

* Eusebius omits the last, and inserts Αμμερης at the beginning as the first.

† Eusebius omits Artabanus, and between Cambyses and Darius places the Magi, with a reign of seven months.

### THE TWENTY-EIGHTH DYNASTY.

| | |
|---|---|
| ΚΗ'. δυναστεια. | |
| Αμυρτεως (Αμυρταιος) Σαϊτης ετη ϛ'. | Amyrteos, the Saïte, 6 years. |

### THE TWENTY-NINTH DYNASTY.

| | |
|---|---|
| ΚΘ'. δυναστεια Μενδησιων βασιλεων δ'. | Of four Mendesian kings. |
| α'. Νεφερειτης (Νεφεριτης) ετη ϛ'. | 1. Nepherites reigned 6 years. |
| β'. Αχωρις ετη ιγ'. | 2. Achoris 13 years. |
| γ'. Ψαμμουθις ετος α'. | 3. Psammuthis 1 year. |
| δ'. Νεφορωτης (Αναφεριτης Νεφεριτης) μηνας δ'. | 4. Nephorotes 4 months. |
| (ε'. Μουθις ετος α'.) | (5. Muthis 1 year.) |
| Ομου ετη κ'. μηνας δ'. | Altogether 20 years and four months. |

### THE THIRTIETH DYNASTY.

| | |
|---|---|
| Τριακοστη δυναστεια Σεβεννυτων βασιλεων τριων. | Of three Sebennyte kings. |
| α'. Νεκτανεβης (Νεκτανεβις) ετη ιη'. | 1. Nectanebes 18 years. |
| β'. Τεως ετη β'. | 2. Teos 2 years. |
| γ'. Νεκτανεβης (Νεκτανεβος) ετη ιη'. | 3. Nectanebes 18 years. |
| Ομου ετη λη'. | Altogether 38 years. |

### THE THIRTY-FIRST DYNASTY.

| | |
|---|---|
| ΛΑ'. δυναστεια Περσων βασιλεων τριων. | Of three Persian kings. |

| | |
|---|---|
| α'. Ωχος εικοστῳ ετει της ἑαυτου βασιλειας Περσων εβασιλευσεν Αιγυπτου ετη ϐ'. | 1. Ochus ruled Persia twenty years, and Egypt 2 years. |
| β'. Αρσης (Αρσης Ωχου) ετη γ'. | 2. Arses reigned 3 years. |
| γ'. Δαρειος ετη δ'. | 3. Darius 4 years. |
| Ομου ετη θ'. | Altogether 9 years. |
| Ομου ͵αν'. | And the whole 1050 years.—*Syncel. Chron.* 73 *to* 78. — *Euseb. Chron.* 16, 17. |

# MANETHO:

## OF THE SHEPHERD KINGS.

ΕΓΕΝΕΤΟ βασιλευς ἡμιν, Τιμαος ονομα, επι τουτου ουκ οιδ᾽ ὁπως ὁ Θεος αντεπνευσεν, και παραδοξως εκ των προς ανατολην μερων, ανθρωποι το γενος ασημοι, καταθαρσησαντες επι την χωραν εστρατευσαν, και ῥαδιως αμαχητι ταυτην κατα κρατος εἱλον. και τους ἡγεμονευσαντας εν αυτη χειρωσαμενοι, το λοιπον τας τε πολεις ωμως ενεπρησαν, και τα ἱερα των θεων κατεσκαψαν. πασι δε τοις επιχωριοις εχθροτατα πως εχρησαντο, τους μεν σφαζοντες, των δε και τα τεκνα και γυναικας εις δουλειαν αγοντες. περας δε και βασιλεα ἑνα εξ αυτων εποιησαν, ᾧ ονομα ην Σαλατις. και οὑτος εν τη Μεμφιδι κατεγινετο, την τε ανω και κατω χωραν δασμολογων, και φρουραν εν τοις επιτηδειοτατοις

We had formerly a king whose name was Timaus. In his time it came to pass, I know not how, that God was displeased with us: and there came up from the East in a strange manner men of an ignoble race, who had the confidence to invade our country, and easily subdued it by their power without a battle. And when they had our rulers in their hands, they burnt our cities, and demolished the temples of the gods, and inflicted every kind of barbarity upon the inhabitants, slaying some, and reducing the wives and children of others to a state of slavery. At length they made one of themselves king, whose name was Salatis: he lived at Memphis, and rendered both the upper and lower regions of Egypt tributary, and stationed garrisons in places which were best adapted for that purpose. But he directed his attention principally to the security καταλειπων τοποις. μαλιστα δε και τα προς ανατολην ησφαλισατο μερη, προορωμενος Ασσυριων, τοτε μειζον ισχυοντων, εσομενην επιθυμιαν της αυτης βασιλειας εφοδου. εὑρων δε εν νομῳ τῳ Σαΐτῃ πολιν επικαιροτατην, κειμενην μεν προς ανατολην του Βουβαττιτου ποταμου, καλουμενην δ' απο τινος αρχαιας θεολογιας Αυαριν, ταυτην εκτισεν τε, και τοις τειχεσιν οχυρωτατην εποιησεν ενοικισας αυτῃ και πληθος ὁπλιτων εις εικοσι και τεσσαρας μυριαδας ανδρων προς φυλακην. ενθαδε κατα θερειαν ηρχετο, τα μεν σιτομετρων και μισθοφοριαν παρεχομενος, τα δε και ταις εξοπλισιαις προς φοβον των εξωθεν επιμελως γυμναζων.

Αρξας δ' εννεακαιδεκα ετη τον βιον ετελευτησαν. Μετα τουτον δε ἑτερος εβασιλευσεν τεσσαρα και τετταρακοντα ετη, καλουμενος Βηων. μεθ' ὁν αλλος Απαχνας, ἑξ και τριακοντα ετη και μηνας ἑπτα. επειτα δε και Αποφις ἑν και ἑξηκοντα, και Ιαννας πεντηκοντα και μηνα ἑνα. επι πασι δε και Ασσις εννεα και τεσσαρακοντα και μηνας δυο. Και οὑτοι μεν ἑξ εν αυτοις εγενηθησαν πρωτοι αρχοντες, πολε-

of the eastern frontier; for he regarded with suspicion the increasing power of the Assyrians, who he foresaw would one day undertake an invasion of the kingdom. And observing in the Saïte nome, upon the east of the Bubastite channel, a city which from some ancient theological reference was called Avaris; and finding it admirably adapted to his purpose, he rebuilt it, and strongly fortified it with walls, and garrisoned it with a force of two hundred and fifty thousand armed men. To this city Salatis repaired in summer time, to collect his tribute, and pay his troops, and to exercise his soldiers in order to strike terror into foreigners.

And Salatis died after a reign of nineteen years: after him reigned Beon forty-four years: and he was succeeded by Apachnas who reigned thirty-six years and seven months: after him reigned Apophis sixty-one years, and Ianias fifty years and one month. After all these reigned Assis forty-nine years and two months. These six were the first rulers amongst them, and during all the period of their dynasty, they made war upon the Egyptians in hope of exterminating the whole race. All this nation was styled μουντες αει και ποθουντες μαλλον της Αιγυπτου εξαραι την ῥιξαν. Εκαλειτο δε το συμπαν αυτων εθνος Ὑκσως, τουτο δε εστι βασιλεις ποιμενες. το γαρ Ὑκ καθ' ἱεραν γλωσσαν βασιλεα σημαινει, το δε Σως ποιμην εστι και ποιμενες κατα την κοινην διαλεκτον, και οὑτω συντιθεμενον γινεται Ὑκσως. τινες δε λεγουσιν αυτους Αραβας ειναι. Τουτους δε τους προκατωνομασμενους βασιλεας τους των ποιμενων καλουμενων, και τους εξ αυτων γενομενους, κρατησαι της Αιγυπτου (φησιν) ετη προς τοις πεντακοσιοις ἑνδεκα.

Hycsos, that is the Shepherd Kings; for the first syllable, Hyc, according to the sacred dialect, denotes a king, and Sos signifies a shepherd, but this according to the vulgar tongue; and of these is compounded the term Hycsos: some say they were Arabians. This people, who were thus denominated Shepherd Kings, and their descendants retained possession of Egypt for the space of five hundred and eleven years.

Μετα ταυτα δε, των εκ της Θεβαΐδος και της αλλης Αιγυπτου βασιλεων γενεσθαι (φησιν) επι τους ποιμενας επαναστασιν, και πολεμον αυτοις συῤῥαγηναι μεγαν και πολυχρονιον. επι δε βασιλεως, ᾡ ονομα ειναι Αλισφραγμουθωσις, ἡττωμενους (φησι) τους ποιμενας ὑπ' αυτου, εκ μεν της αλλης Αιγυπτου πασης εκπεσειν, κατακλεισθηναι δ' εις τοπον, αρουρων εχοντα μυριων την περιμετρον. Αυαριν ονομα τῳ τοπῳ. Τουτον (φησιν ὁ Μανεθων) ἁπαντα, τειχει τε μεγαλῳ και ισχυρῳ περιβαλειν τους ποιμενας, ὁπως την τε κτησιν ἁπασαν εχωσιν εν οχυρῳ, και την λειαν την ἑαυτων.

After these things he relates that the kings of Thebaïs and of the other parts of Egypt, made an insurrection against the Shepherds, and that a long and mighty war was carried on between them, till the Shepherds were subdued by a king whose name was Alisphragmuthosis, and were by him driven out of the rest of Egypt, and hemmed within a place containing ten thousand acres, which was called Avaris. All this tract (says Manetho) the Shepherds surrounded with a vast and strong wall, that they might retain all their possessions and their prey within a hold of strength.

Τον δε Αλισφραγμουθωσεως υἱον Θουμμωσιν επιχειρησαι μεν αυτους δια πολιορκιας ἑλειν κατα κρατος, οκτω και τεσσαρακοντα μυριασι προσεδρευσαντα τοις τειχεσιν· επει δε της πολιορκιας απεγνω, ποιησασθαι συμβασεις, ἱνα την Αιγυπτον εκλιποντες ὁποι βουλονται παντες αβλαβεις απελθωσι. τους δε επι ταις ὁμολογιαις πανοικεσια μετα των κτησεων ουκ ελαττους μυριαδων οντας εικοσι και τεσσαρων απο της Αιγυπτου την ερημον εις Συριαν ὁδοιπορησαι. φοβουμενους δε την Ασσυριων δυναστειαν, τοτε γαρ εκεινους της Ασιας κρατειν, εν τῃ νυν Ιουδαια καλουμενῃ πολιν οικοδομησαμενους τοσαυταις μυριασιν ανθρωπων αρκεσουσαν, Ἱεροσολυμα ταυτην ονομασαι.

(Εν αλλῃ δε τινι βιβλῳ των Αιγυπτιακων Μανεθων) Τουτο (φησιν) εθνος τους καλουμενους ποιμενας, αιχμαλωτους εν ταις ἱεραις αυτων βιβλοις γεγραφθαι.

Μετα το εξελθειν εξ Αιγυπτου τον λαον των ποιμενων εις Ἱεροσολυμα, ὁ εκβαλων αυτους εξ Αιγυπτου βασιλευς Τεθμωσις, εβασιλευσεν μετα ταυτα ετη εικοσι πεντε και μηνας τεσσαρας, και ετελευτησεν, και παρελαβε την αρχην αυτου

And Thummosis, the son of Alisphragmuthosis, endeavoured to force them by a siege, and beleaguered the place with a body of four hundred and eighty thousand men; but at the moment when he despaired of reducing them by siege, they agreed to a capitulation, that they would leave Egypt, and should be permitted to go out without molestation wheresoever they pleased. And, according to this stipulation, they departed from Egypt with all their families and effects, in number not less than two hundred and forty thousand, and bent their way through the desert towards Syria. But as they stood in fear of the Assyrians, who had then dominion over Asia, they built a city in that country which is now called Judæa, of sufficient size to contain this multitude of men, and named it Jerusalem.

(In another book of the Egyptian histories Manetho says) That this people, who are here called Shepherds, in their sacred books were also styled Captives.

After the departure of this nation of Shepherds to Jerusalem, Tethmosis, the king of Egypt who drove them out, reigned twenty-five years and four months, and then died: after him his son Chebron took the government into his hands for thirteen years; after him reigned Amenoυἱὸς Χεβρων ετη δεκατρια. μεθ' ὃν Αμεναφις εικοσι και μηνας ἑπτα. του δε αδελφη Αμεσσης εικοσι ἑν και μηνας εννεα. της δε Μηφρης δωδεκα και μηνας εννεα. του δε Μηφραμουθωσις εικοσι πεντε και μηνας δεκα. του δε Θμωσις εννεα και μηνας οκτω. του δε Αμενωφις τριακοντα και μηνας δεκα. του δε Ωρος τριακοντα ἑξ και μηνας πεντε. του δε θυγατηρ Ακεγχρης δωδεκα και μηνα ἑνα. της δε Ραθωτις αδελφος εννεα. του δε Ακεγχηρης δωδεκα και μηνας πεντε. του δε Ακεγχηρης ἑτερος δωδεκα και μηνας τρεις. του δε Αρμαϊς τεσσαρα και μηνα ἑνα. του δε Ραμεσσης ἑν και μηνας τεσσαρας. του δε Αρμεσσης Μιαμμου εξηκοντα ἑξ και μηνας δυο. του δε Αμενωφις δεκα και εννεα και μηνας ἑξ. του δε Σεθωσις, και Ραμεσσης, ἱππικην και ναυτικην εχων δυναμιν.

Οὗτος τον μεν αδελφον Αρμαϊν επιτροπον της Αιγυπτου κατεστησεν, και πασαν μεν αυτῳ την αλλην βασιλικην περιεθηκεν εξουσιαν, μονον δε ενετειλατο διαδημα μη φορειν, μηδε την βασιλιδα μητερα τε των τεκνων αδικειν, απεχεσθαι δε και των αλλων βασιλικων παλλακιδων. αυτος δε επι

phis for twenty years and seven months: then his sister Amesses twenty-one years and nine months: she was succeeded by Mephres, who reigned twelve years and nine months: after him Mephramnthosis twenty-five years and ten months: then Thmosis reigned nine years and eight months; after whom Amenophis thirty years and ten months: then Orus thirty-six years and five months: then his daughter Acenchres twelve years and one month: after her Rathotis nine years: then Acencheres twelve years and five months: another Acencheres twelve years and three months: after him Armaïs four years and one month: after him reigned Ramesses one year and four months: then Armesses the son of Miammous sixty-six years and two months: after him Amenophis nineteen years and six months: and he was succeeded by Sethosis who is called Ramesses, he maintained an army of cavalry and a naval force.

This king (Sethosis) appointed his brother Armaïs his viceroy over Egypt: he also invested him with all the other authority of a king, but with these restrictions; that he should not wear the diadem, nor interfere with the queen, the mother of his children, nor abuse the royal concubines. Sethosis then made an expedition against Cyprus and Phœnicia, and waged

Κυπρον και Φοινικην και παλιν Ασσυριους τε και Μηδους ϛρατευσας, άπαντας, τους μεν δορατι, τους δε αμαχητι, φοϐῳ δε της πολλης δυναμεως, ὑποχειριους ελαϐε. και μεγα φρονησας επι ταις ευπραγιαις, ετι και θαρσαλεωτερον επορευετο, τας προς ανατολας πολεις τε και χωρας καταστρεφομενος.

war with the Assyrians and Medes; and he subdued them all, some by force of arms, and others without a blow, by the mere terror of his power. And being puffed up with his success, he advanced still more confidently, and overthrew the cities, and subdued the countries of the East.

Χρονου τε ἱκανου γεγονοτος, Αρμαΐς ὁ καταλειφθεις εν Αιγυπτῳ, παντα τουμπαλιν, οἷς αδελφος παρῄνει μη ποιειν, αδεως επραττεν. και γαρ την βασιλιδα βιαιως εσχεν, και ταις αλλαις παλλακισιν αφειδως διετελει χρωμενος. πειθομενος δε ὑπο των φιλων διαδημα εφορει, και αντηρε τῳ αδελφῳ.

But Armaïs, who was left in Egypt, took advantage of the opportunity, and fearlessly committed all those acts which his brother had enjoined him not to do: he violated the queen, and continued an unrestrained intercourse with the rest, and at the persuasion of his friends he assumed the diadem, and openly opposed his brother.

Ὁ δε τεταγμενος επι των ἱερων της Αιγυπτου, γραψας βιϐλιον επεμψε τῳ Σεθωσει, δηλων αυτῳ παντα, και ὅτι αντηρεν ὁ αδελφος αυτου Αρμαΐς. παραχρημα ουν ὑπεστρεψεν εις Πηλουσιον, και εκρατησεν της ιδιας βασιλειας. ἡ δε χωρα εκληθη απο του αυτου ονοματος Αιγυπτος. λεγει γαρ ὅτι ὁ μεν Σεθωσις εκαλειτο Αιγυπτος, Αρμαΐς δε ὁ Αδελφος αυτου Δαναος.

But the ruler over the priests of Egypt sent to Sethosis, and informed him of what had happened, and how his brother had set himself up in opposition to his power. Upon this Sethosis immediately returned to Pelusium, and recovered his kingdom. The country of Egypt took its name from Sethosis, who was called also Ægyptus, as was his brother Armaïs known by the name of Danaus.—*Joseph. contr. App.* lib. I. c. 14, 15.

## OF THE ISRAELITES.

Τουτον (Αμενωφιν) επιθυμησαι θεων γενεσθαι θεατην, ὥσπερ Ωρος εἷς των προ αυτου βεβασιλευκοτων· ανενεγκειν δε την επιθυμιαν ὁμωνυμῳ μεν αυτῳ Αμενωφει, πατρος δε Παπιος οντι, θειας δε δοκουντι μετεσχηκεναι φυσεως, κατα τε σοφιαν και προγνωσιν των εσομενων. ειπειν ουν αυτῳ τουτον τον ὁμωνυμον, ὅτι δυνησεται θεους ιδειν, ει καθαραν απο τε λεπρων και των αλλων μιαρων ανθρωπων την χωραν ἅπασαν ποιησειεν.

This king (Amenophis) was desirous of beholding the gods, as Orus, one of his predecessors in the kingdom, had seen them. And he communicated his desire to a priest of the same name with himself, Amenophis, the son of Papis, who seemed to partake of the divine nature, both in his wisdom and knowledge of futurity: and Amenophis returned him answer, that he might behold the gods, if he would cleanse the country of all lepers and other unclean persons that were in it.

Ἡσθεντα δε τον βασιλεα, παντας τους τα σωματα λελωβημενους εκ της Αιγυπτου συναγαγειν· γενεσθαι δε του πληθους μυριαδας οκτω· και τουτους εις τας λιθοτομιας τας εν τῳ προς ανατολην μερει του Νειλου εμβαλειν αυτον, ὅπως εργαζοιντο και των αλλων Αιγυπτιων οἱ εγκεχωρισμενοι. ειναι δε τινας εν αυτοις και των λογιων ἱερεων (φησι,) λεπρα συγκεχυμενους. τον δε Αμενωφιν εκεινον, τον σοφον και μαντικον ανδρα, ὑποδεισθαι προς αυτον τε και τον βασιλεα χολον των θεων, ει βιασθεντες οφθησον-

Well pleased with this information, the king gathered together out of the land of Egypt all that laboured under any defect in body, to the amount of eighty thousand, and sent them to the quarries, which are situate on the east side of the Nile, that they might work in them and be separated from the rest of the Egyptians. And (he says) there were among them some learned priests who were affected with leprosy. And Amenophis the wise man and prophet, fearful lest the vengeance of the gods should fall both on himself and on the king, if it should appear that violence had been offered them, added this also ται. και προσθεμενον ειπειν, ὁτι συμμαχησουσι τινες τοις μιαροις, και της Αιγυπτου κρατησουσιν επ' ετη δεκατρια. μη τολμησαι μεν αυτον ειπειν ταυτα τῳ βασιλει, γραφην δε καταλιποντα περι παντων ἑαυτον ανελειν. εν αθυμιᾳ δε ειναι τον βασιλεα.

in a prophetic spirit;—that certain people would come to the assistance of these polluted wretches, and would subdue Egypt, and hold it in possession for thirteen years. These tidings however he dared not to communicate to the king, but left in writing an account of what should come to pass, and destroyed himself, at which the king was fearfully distressed.

(Κᾳπειτα κατα λεξιν οὑτω γεγραφεν). Των δε ταις λατομιαις ὡς χρονος ἱκανος διηλθεν ταλαιπωρουντων, αξιωθεις ὁ βασιλευς, ἱνα προς καταλυσιν αυτοις και σκεπην απομεριση την τοτε των ποιμενων ερημωθεισαν πολιν, Αυαριν συνεχωρησεν. εστι δε ἡ πολις κατα την θεολογιαν ανωθεν Τυφωνιος.

(After which he writes thus, word for word:) When those that were sent to work in the quarries had continued for some time in that miserable state, the king was petitioned to set apart for their habitation and protection the city Avaris, which had been left desolate by the Shepherds; and he granted them their desire: now this city, according to the theology above, is a Typhonian city.

Οἱ δε εις ταυτην εισελθοντες, και τον τοπον τουτον εις αποστασιν εχοντες, ἡγεμονα αὑτων λεγομενον τινα των Ἡλιοπολιτων ἱερων Οσαρσιφον εστησαντο. και τουτῳ πειθαρχησοντες εν πασιν ὡρκομοτησαν· ὁ δε πρωτον μεν αυτοις νομον εθετο, μητε προσκυνειν θεους, μητε των μαλιστα εν Αιγυπτῳ θεμιστευομενων ἱερων ζωων απεχεσθαι μηδενος, παντα τε θυειν και αναλουν· συναπτεσθαι δε μηδενι πλην των συνωμοσμενων. τοιαυτα δε

When these men had taken possession of the city, and found it well adapted for a revolt, they appointed over themselves a ruler out of the priests of Heliopolis, one whose name was Osarsiph, and they bound themselves by oath that they would be obedient. Osarsiph then, in the first place enacted this law, that they should neither worship the gods, nor abstain from any of those sacred animals which the Egyptians hold in the highest veneration, but sacrifice and slay them all, and that they should connect themselves with none but νομοθετησας, και πλειστα αλλα, μαλιστα τοις Αιγυπτιοις εθισμοις εναντιουμενα, εκελευσεν πολυχειρια τα της πολεως επισκευαζειν τειχη, και προς πολεμον έτοιμους γινεσθαι τον προς Αμενωφιν τον βασιλεα. αυτος δε προσλαβομενος μεθ' έαυτου και των αλλων ἱερεων και συμμεμιασμενων, επεμψε πρεσβεις προς τους ὑπο Τεθμωσιως απελαθεντας ποιμενας, εις πολιν την καλουμενην Ἱεροσολυμα και τα καθ' έαυτον και τους αλλους τους συνατιμασθεντας δηλωσας, ηξιου συνεπιστρατευειν ὁμοθυμαδον επ' Αιγυπτον. επαξειν μεν ουν αυτους επηγγειλατο, πρωτον μεν εις Αυαριν την προγονικην αυτων πατριδα, και τα επιτηδεια τοις οχλοις παρεξειν αφθονως, ὑπερμαχησεσθαι δε οτε δεοι, και ῥαδιως ὑποχειριον αυτοις την χωραν ποιησειν. οἱ δε ὑπερχαρεις γενομενοι παντες προθυμως εις εικοσι μυριαδας ανδρων συνεξωρμησαν, και μετ' ου πολυ ἡκον εις Αυαριν.

such as were of that confederacy. When he had made such laws as these, and many others of a tendency directly in opposition to the customs of the Egyptians, he gave orders that they should employ the multitude of hands in rebuilding the walls about the city, and hold themselves in readiness for war with Amenophis the king, whilst he took into his confidence and counsels some others of the priests and unclean persons: and he sent ambassadors to the city called Jerusalem, to those Shepherds who had been expelled by Tethmosis, whereby he informed them of the affairs of himself and of the others who had been treated in the same ignominious manner, and requested they would come with one consent to his assistance in this war against Egypt. He also promised in the first place to reinstate them in their ancient city and country Avaris, and provide a plentiful maintenance for their host, and fight for them as occasion might require; and informed them that they could easily reduce the country under dominion. The Shepherds received this message with the greatest joy, and quickly mustered to the number of two hundred thousand men, and came up to Avaris.

Αμενωφις δ' ὁ των Αιγυπτιων βασιλευς, ὡς επυθετο τα κατα την εκεινων εφοδον, ου

Now Amenophis the king of Egypt, when he was informed of their invasion, was in great consternation, μετριως συνεχυθη, της παρ' Αμενωφεως του Παπιος μνησθεις προδηλωσεως. και προτερον συναγαγων πληθος Αιγυπτιων, και βουλευσαμενος μετα των εν τουτοις ἡγεμονων, τα τε ἱερα ζωα τα πρωτα μαλιστα εν τοις ἱεροις τιμωμενα ὡς γ' ἑαυτον μετεπεμψατο, και τοις κατα μερος ἱερευσιν παρηγγειλεν, ὡς ασφαλεστατα των θεων συγκρυψαι τα ξοανα. τον δε υἱον Σεθων τον και Ραμεσσην απο Ραμψεως του πατρος ωνομασμενον πενταετη οντα, εξεθετο προς τον ἑαυτου φιλον. αυτος δε διαβας τοις αλλοις Αιγυπτιοις, ουσιν εις τριακοντα μυριαδας ανδρων μαχιμωτατων, και τοις πολεμιοις απαντησασιν ου συνεβαλεν· αλλα μελλειν θεομαχειν νομισας, παλινδρομησας ἡκεν εις Μεμφιν. αναλαβων τε τον τε Απιν, και τα αλλα τα εκεισε μεταπεμφθεντα ἱερα ζωα, ευθυς εις Αιθιοπιαν συν ἁπαντι τῳ στολῳ και πληθει των Αιγυπτιων ανηχθη. χαριτι γαρ ην αυτῳ ὑποχειριος ὁ των Αιθιοπων βασιλευς· ὁθεν ὑποδεξαμενος, και τους οχλους παντας ὑπολαβων οἱς εσχεν ἡ χωρα των προς ανθρωπινην τροφην επιτηδειων, και πολεις και κωμας προς την των πε-

remembering the prophecy of Amenophis, the son of Papis, and he assembled the armies of the Egyptians, and took counsel with the leaders, and commanded the sacred animals to be brought to him, especially those which were held in the greatest veneration in the temples, and particularly charged the priests to conceal the images of their gods with the utmost care. And his son Sethos, who was also called Ramesses from his father Rampses, being but five years old he committed to the protection of a friend. And he marched with the rest of the Egyptians being three hundred thousand warriors, against the enemy, who advanced to meet him; but he did not attack them, thinking it would be to wage war against the gods, but he returned, and came again to Memphis, where he took Apis and the other sacred animals he had sent for, and retreated immediately into Ethiopia together with all his army, and all the multitude of the Egyptians: for the king of Ethiopia was under obligations to him, wherefore he received him kindly, and took care of all the multitude that was with him, while the country supplied all that was necessary for their food. He also allotted to him cities and villages during his exile, which was to continue from its beginning during the predestined thirteen years. Moreπρωμενων τρισκαιδεκα ετων απο της αρχης αυτου εκπτωσιν αυταρκεις, ουκ ἡττον γε και στρατοπεδον Αιθιοπικον προς φυλακην επεταξε τοις παρ' Αμενωφεως του βασιλεως επι των ὁριων της Αιγυπτου.

Και τα μεν κατα την Αιθιοπιαν τοιαυτα. οἱ δε Σολυμιται κατελθοντες, συν τοις μιαροις των Αιγυπτιων οὑτως ανοσιως τοις ανθρωποις προσηνεχθησαν, ὡστε την των προειρημενων κρατησιν χειριστην φαινεσθαι, τοις τοτε τα τουτων ασεβηματα θεωμενοις. και γαρ ου μονον πολεις και κωμας ενεπρησαν, ουδε ἱεροσυλουντες, ουδε λυμαινομενοι ξοανα θεων ηρκουντο, αλλα και τοις αυτοις οπτανιοις των σεβαστευομενων ἱερων ζωων χρωμενοι διετελουν, και θυτας και σφαγεις τουτων ἱερεις και προφητας ηναγκαζον γινεσθαι, και γυμνους εξεβαλον. λεγεται δ' ὁτι την πολιτειαν και τους νομους αυτοις καταβαλλομενος ἱερευς, το γενος Ἡλιουπολιτης, ονομα Οσαρσιφ, απο του εν Ἡλιου πολει θεου Οσιρεως, ὡς μετεβη εις τουτο το γενος, μετετεθη τουνομα και προσηγορευθη Μωϋσης.

over he pitched a camp for an Ethiopian army upon the borders of Egypt, as a protection to king Amenophis.

While such was the state of things in Ethiopia, the people of Jerusalem, having come down with the unclean of the Egyptians, treated the inhabitants with such barbarity, that those who witnessed their impieties believed that their joint sway was more execrable than that which the Shepherds had formerly exercised: for they not only set fire to the cities and villages, but committed every kind of sacrilege, and destroyed the images of the gods, and roasted and fed upon those sacred animals that were worshipped; and having compelled the priests and prophets to kill and sacrifice them, they cast them naked out of the country. It is said also that the priest, who ordained their polity and laws, was by birth of Heliopolis, and his name Osarsiph, from Osiris the god of Heliopolis: but that when he went over to these people his name was changed, and he was called Moÿses.—*Joseph. contr. App.* lib. I. c. 26.

## OF THE ISRAELITES.

(Λεγει δε ὁ Μανεθων παλιν.) 'Οτι μετα ταυτα επηλθεν ὁ Αμενωφις απο Αιθιοπιας μετα μεγαλης δυναμεως, και ὁ υἱος αυτου Ραμψης και αυτος εχων δυναμιν· και συμβαλοντες οἱ δυο τοις ποιμεσι και τοις μιαροις, ενικησαν αυτους, και πολλους αποκτειναντες εδιωξαν αυτους αχρι των ὁριων της Συριας.

(Manetho again says:) After this Amenophis returned from Ethiopia with a great force, and Rampses also, his son, with other forces, and encountering the Shepherds and the unclean people, they defeated them and slew multitudes of them, and pursued them to the bounds of Syria. — *Joseph. contr. App.* lib. I. c. 27.

# ERATOSTHENES'

## CANON OF THE KINGS OF THEBES.

ΠΡΩΤΟΣ εβασιλευσεν Μινης Θηβινιτης Θηβαιος, ὁ ἑρμηνευεται Διονιος· εβασιλευσεν ετη ξβ'. του δε κοσμου ην ετος ,ϡπ'.

The first who reigned was Mines the Thebinite, the Thebæan; which is by interpretation Dionius. He reigned sixty-two years, and lived in the year of the world 2900.

Θηβαιων δευτερος εβασιλευσεν Αθωθης υἱος Μινεως ετη νθ'. οὑτος ἑρμηνευεται Ἑρμογενης· ετος του κοσμου ,ϡξβ'.

The 2nd of the Theban kings reigned Athothes the son of Mines, 59 years. He is called by interpretation Hermogenes. In the year of the world 2962.

Θηβαιων Αιγυπτιων τριτος εβασιλευσεν Αθωθης ὁμωνυμος ετη λβ'. του δε κοσμου ην ετος, ,γκα'.

The 3rd of the Theban Egyptian kings was Athothes, of the same name, 32 years. In the year of the world 3021.

Θηβαιων εβασιλευσεν δ'. Διαβιης υἱος Αθωσεως ετη ιθ'. οὑτος ἑρμηνευεται Φιλεστερος· του δε κοσμου ην ετος, ,γνγ'.

The 4th of the Theban kings was Diabies the son of Athothes, 19 years. By interpretation he is called Philesteros. In the year of the world 3053.

Θηβαιων εβασιλευσεν ε'. Πεμφως υἱος Αθωθου ὁ εστιν Ἡρακλειδης ετη ιη'. του δε κοσμου ην ετος ,γοβ'.

The 5th of the Theban kings was Pemphos, the son of Athothes, who is called Heraclides. He reigned 18 years. In the year of the world 3072.

Θηβαιων Αιγυπτιων εβασιλευσεν ϛ'. Τοιγαρ Αμαχος

The 6th of the Theban Egyptian kings was Tœgar Amachus Mom-

Μομχειρι Μεμφιτης ετη οθ΄. οὗτος ἑρμηνευεται της ανδρος περισσομελης· του δε κοσμου ην ετος ,γϟ΄.

chiri, the Memphite, who is called a man redundant in his members, 79 years and A. M. 3090.

Θηβαιων Αιγυπτιων εβασιλευσεν ζ΄. Στοιχος ὁ υἱος αυτου, ὁ εστιν Αρης αναισθητος, ετη ϛ΄. του δε κοσμου ην ετος, ,γρξθ΄.

The 7th of the Theban Egyptian kings, Stœchus his son, who is Ares the senseless, reigned 6 years, A. M. 3169.

Θηβαιων Αιγυπτιων εβασιλευσεν ογδοος Γοσορμιης, ὁ εστιν Ετησιπαντος ετη λ΄. του δε κοσμου ην ετος ,γροε΄.

The 8th of the Theban Egyptian kings Gosormies, who is called Etesipantus, reigned 30 years, and A. M. 3175.

Θηβαιων Αιγυπτιων εβασιλευσεν θ΄. Μαρης υἱος αυτου, ὁ εστιν Ἡλιοδωρος ετη κϛ΄. του κοσμου ην ετος γσε΄.

The 9th of the Theban Egyptian kings Mares, his son, who is called Heliodorus, 26 years, and A. M. 3205.

Θηβαιων Αιγυπτιων ι΄. εβασιλευσεν Ανωΰφης, ὁ εστιν υἱος επικοινος ετη κ΄. του κοσμου ην ετος, ,γσλα΄.

The 10th of the Theban Egyptian kings Anoÿphes, which signifies a common son, reigned 20 years, and A. M. 3231.

Θηβαιων Αιγυπτιων ια΄. εβασιλευσεν Σιριος, ὁ εστιν κορρης, ὡς δε ἑτεροι Αβασκαντος ετη ιη΄. του δε κοσμου ην ετος, ,γσνα΄.

The 11th of the Theban Egyptian kings Sirius, which signifies the son of the cheek, but according to others Abascantus reigned 18 years, and A. M. 3251.

Θηβαιων Αιγυπτιων ιβ΄. εβασιλευσεν Χνουβος Γνευρος, ὁ εστιν Χρυσης Χρυσου υἱος ετη κβ΄. του δε κοσμου ην ετος, ,γσξθ΄.

The 12th of the Theban Egyptian kings reigned Chnubus Gneurus, which is Chryses the son of Chryses, 22 years, A. M. 3269.

Θηβαιων Αιγυπτιων ιγ΄. εβασιλευσεν Ρανωσις, ὁ εστιν αχρικρατωρ ετη ιγ΄. του δε κοσμου ην ετος, ,γσϟα΄.

The 13th of the Theban Egyptian kings reigned Ranosis, which is Archicrator, 13 years, A. M. 3291.

Θηβαιων Αιγυπτιων ιδ΄.

The 14th of the Theban Egyptian

εβασιλευσεν Βιϊρις ετη ι'. του δε κοσμου ην ετος ,γτδ'.

kings reigned Biyris, 10 years, A. M. 3304.

Θηβαιων βασιλεων ιε'. εβασιλευσεν Σαωφις Κωμαστης, κατα δε ενιους Χρηματιστης ετη κθ'. του δε κοσμου ην ετος ,γτιδ'.

The 15th of the Theban kings Saophis Comastes, or, according to some, Chrematistes, reigned 29 years, and A. M. 3314.

Θηβαιων ις'. εβασιλευσεν Σενσαωφις β'. ετη κζ'. του δε κοσμου ην ετος ,γτμγ'.

The 16th of the Theban kings Sensaophis the second, reigned 27 years, A. M. 3343.

Θηβαιων εβασιλευσεν Μοσχερις Ἡλιοδοτος ετη λα'. του δε κοσμου ην ετος ,γτο'.

The 17th of the Theban kings, Moscheris Heliodotus, reigned 31 years, A. M. 3370.

Θηβαιων ιη'. εβασιλευσεν Μουσθις ετη λγ'. του δε κοσμου ην ετος ,γυα'.

The 18th of the Theban kings, Musthis, reigned 33 years, A. M. 3401.

Θηβαιων ιθ'. εβασιλευσεν Παμμος Αρχονδης ετη λε'. του δε κοσμου ην ετος ,γυλδ'.

The 19th of the Theban kings, Pammus Archondes, reigned 35 years, A. M. 3434.

Θηβαιων κ'. εβασιλευσεν Απαππους μεγιστος, οὗτος ὥς φασιν παρα ὥραν μιαν εβασιλευσεν ετη ρ'. του δε κοσμου ην ετος ,γυξθ'.

The 20th of the Theban kings, Apaphus Maximus, is said to have reigned 100 years with the exception of one hour, A. M. 3469.

Θηβαιων κα'. εβασιλευσεν Αχεσκος Οκαρας ετος α'. του δε κοσμου ην ετος ,γφξθ'.

The 21st of the Theban kings, Achescus Ocaras, reigned one year, A. M. 3569.

Θηβαιων κβ'. εβασιλευσεν Νιτωκρις αντι του ανδρος, ὅ εστιν Αθηνα Νικηφορος, ετη ς'. του δε κοσμου ην ετος ,γφο'.

The 22nd of the Theban sovereigns was Nitocris, instead of her husband, she is Athena Nicephorus, and reigned 6 years, A. M. 3570.

Θηβαιων κγ'. εβασιλευσεν Μυρταιος Αμμωνοδοτος ετη κβ'. του δε κοσμου ην ετος ,γφος'.

The 23rd of the Theban kings, Myrtæus Ammonodotus, reigned 22 years, A. M. 3576.

Θηβαιων κδ'. εβασιλευσεν Θυοσιμαρης κραταιος, ὁ εστιν

The 24th of the Theban kings, Thyosimares the robust, who is called ἥλιος, ετη ιβ'. του δε κοσμου ην ετος ,γφϟη'.

the sun, reigned 12 years, and A. M. 3598.

Θηβαιων κε'. εβασιλευσεν Θινιλλος, ὁ εστιν αυξησας το πατριον κρατος ετη η'. του δε κοσμου ην ετος ,γχι'.

The 25th of the Theban kings, Thinillus, which is the augmenter of country's strength, reigned 8 years, A. M. 3610.

Θηβαιων κϛ'. εβασιλευσεν Σεμφρουκρατης, ὁ εστιν Ἡρακλης Ἁρποκρατης ετη ιη'. του δε κοσμου ετος ,γχιη'.

The 26th of the Theban kings, Semphrucrates, who is Hercules Harpocrates, reigned 18 years, A. M. 3618.

Θηβαιων κζ'. εβασιλευσεν Χουθηρ Ταυρος τυραννος ετη ζ'. του δε κοσμου ,γχλϛ'.

The 27th of the Theban kings, Chuther Taurus the tyrant, 7 years, A. M. 3636.

Θηβαιων κη'. εβασιλευσεν Μευρης Φιλοσκορος ετη ιβ'. του δε κοσμου ,γχμγ'.

The 28th of the Theban kings, Meures Philoscorus, reigned 12 years, A. M. 3643.

Θηβαιων κθ'. εβασιλευσεν Χωμαεφθα κοσμος Φιληφαιστος ετη ια'. του δε κοσμου ,γχνε'.

The 29th of the Theban kings, Chomaephtha Cosmus Philephæstus, reigned 11 years, A. M. 3655.

Θηβαιων λ'. εβασιλευσεν Αγκουνιος Οχυτυραννος ετη ξ'. του δε κοσμου ,γχξϛ'.

The 30th of the Theban kings, Ancunius Ochytyrannus, reigned 60 years, A. M. 3666.

Θηβαιων λα'. εβασιλευσεν Πενταθυρις ετη μβ'. του δε κοσμου ,γψκϛ'.

The 31st of the Theban kings, Penteathyris, reigned 42 years, A. M. 3726.

Θηβαιων λβ'. εβασιλευσεν Σταμενεμης β'. ετη κγ'. του δε κοσμου ,γψξη'.

The 32nd of the Theban kings, Stamenemes the second, reigned 23 years, A. M. 3768.

Θηβαιων λγ'. εβασιλευσεν Σιστοσιχερμης Ἡρακλεος κρατος ετη νε'. του δε κοσμου, ,γψϟα'.

The 33rd of the Theban kings, Sistosichermes, the strength of Hercules, reigned 55 years, A. M. 3791.

Θηβαιων λδ'. εβασιλευσεν Μαρις ετη μγ'. του δε κοσμου ,γωμϛ'.

The 34th of the Theban kings, Maris, reigned 43 years, A. M. 3846.

Θηβαιων λε΄. εβασιλευσεν Σιφωας, ὁ και Ἑρμης υἱος Ἡφαιστου, ετη ε΄. του δε κοσμου, ,γωπθ΄.

The 35th of the Theban kings, Siphoas, which is Hermes the son of Hephæstus, reigned 5 years, A. M. 3889.

Θηβαιων λϛ΄. εβασιλευσεν . . . . . . ετη ιδ΄. του δε κοσμου ,γωϟδ΄.

The 36th of the Theban kings, . . . . . . reigned 14 years, A. M. 3894.

Θηβαιων λζ΄. εβασιλευσεν Φρουρων, ητοι Νειλος, ετη ε΄. του δε κοσμου ,γϡη΄.

The 37th of the Theban kings, Phruron, which is Nilus, reigned 5 years, A. M. 3908.

Θηβαιων λη΄. εβασιλευσεν Αμουθανταιος ετη ξγ΄. του δε κοσμου ,γϡιγ΄.

The 38th of the Theban kings, Amuthantæus, reigned 63 years, A.M. 3913.—*Syncel. Chron.* 91. 96. 101. 104. 109. 123. 147.

# THE FRAGMENTS

OF

# THE TYRIAN ANNALS:

FROM

DIUS AND MENANDER.

# THE TYRIAN ANNALS:

## FROM DIUS.

### OF HIRAM.

ΑΒΙΒΑΛΟΥ τελευτησαντος, ὁ υἱος αυτου Εἰρωμος εβασιλευσεν· οὗτος τα προς ἀνατολας μερη της πολεως προσεχωσεν, και μειζον το αστυ πεποιηκεν, και του Ολυμπιου Διος το ἱερον καθ' ἑαυτο ον εν νησῳ, χωσας τον μεταξυ τοπον, συνηψε τῃ πολει, και χρυσοις αναθημασιν εκοσμησεν· αναβας δε εις τον Λιβανον ὑλοτομησε προς την των ναων κατασκευην. τον δε τυραννουντα Ἱεροσολυμων Σολομωνα πεμψαι (φασι) προς τον Εἰρωμον αινιγματα, και παρ' αυτου λαβειν αξιουν· τον δε μη δυνηθεντα διακριναι, τῳ λυσαντι χρηματα αποτινειν. ὁμολογησαντα δε τον Εἰρωμον, και μη δυνηθεντα λυσαι τα αινιγματα, πολλα των χρηματων

Upon the death of Abibalus his son Hiromus succeeded to the kingdom. He raised the eastern parts of the city, and enlarged it; and joined to it the temple of Jupiter Olympius, which stood before upon an island, by filling up the intermediate space: and he adorned that temple with donations of gold: and he went up into Libanus to cut timber for the construction of the temples. And it is said that Solomon, king of Jerusalem, sent enigmas to Hiromus, and desired others in return, with a proposal that whichsoever of the two was unable to solve them, should forfeit money to the other. Hiromus agreed to the proposal, but was unable to solve the enigmas, and paid a large sum as a forfeit. And it is said that one Abdemonus, a Tyrian, solved the enigmas, and proposed others εις το επιζημιον αναλωσαι. ειτα δε Αβδημονον τινα Τυριον ανδρα τα προτεθεντα λυσαι και αυτον αλλα προβαλειν· ἁ μη λυσαντα τον Σολομωνα, πολλα τῳ Ειρωμῳ προσαποτισαι χρηματα.

which Solomon was not able to unriddle, for which he repaid the fine to Hiromus.—*Joseph. contr. App.* lib. I. c. 17.—*Syncel. Chron.* 182.

# THE TYRIAN ANNALS:

## FROM MENANDER.

---

### OF HIRAM.

ΤΕΛΕΥΤΗΣΑΝΤΟΣ δε Αβιβαλου, διεδεξατο την βασιλειαν ὁ υἱος αυτου Ειρωμος, ὃς βιωσας ετη πεντηκοντα τρια εβασιλευσεν ετη τριακοντα τεσσαρα. οὗτος εχωσε τον Ευρυχωρον, τον τε χρυσουν κιονα εν τοις του Διος ανεθηκεν· ετι τε ὕλην ξυλων απελθων εκοψεν, απο του λεγομενου ορους Λιβανου, κεδρινα ξυλα εις τας των ἱερων στεγας. καθελων τε τα αρχαια ἱερα, καινους ναους ᾠκοδομησε, το τε του Ἡρακλεους, και της Ασταρτης τεμενος ανιερευσεν, και το μεν του Ἡρακλεους πρωτον εποιησατο εν τῳ Περιτιῳ μηνι, ειτα το της Ασταρτης, ὁποτε Τιτυοις επεστρατευσεν, μη αποδιδουσι τους φορους. οὓς και ὑποταξας

AFTER the death of Abibalus, Hiromus his son succeeded him in his kingdom, and reigned thirty-four years, having lived fifty-three. He laid out that part of the city which is called Eurychoron: and consecrated the golden column which is in the temple of Jupiter. And he went up into the forest on the mountain called Libanus, to fell cedars for the roofs of the temples: and having demolished the ancient temples, he rebuilt them, and consecrated the fanes of Hercules and Astarte: he constructed that of Hercules first, in the month Peritius; then that of Astarte, when he had overcome the Tityans who had refused to pay their tribute: and when he had reduced them he returned. In his time was a certain young man named Abdemonus, who used to solve the problems which were propounded ἑαυτῳ παλιν ανεστρεψεν. επι τουτου δε τις ην Αβδημονος παις νεωτερος, ὁς ενικα τα προβληματα, ἁ επετασσε Σολομων ὁ Ἱεροσολυμων βασιλευς.

to him by Solomon king of Jerusalem. —*Joseph. contr. App.* lib. I. c. 18.—*Joseph. Antiq. Jud.* lib. VIII. c. 5.

## OF THE SUCCESSORS OF HIRAM.

Τελευτησαντος Εἰρωμου διεδεξατο την βασιλειαν Βαλεαζαρος ὁ υἱος, ὁς, βιωσας ετη τεσσαρακοντα τρια, εβασιλευσεν ετη ἑπτα. μετα τουτον Αβδαστρατος ὁ αυτου υἱος, βιωσας ετη εικοσι εννεα, εβασιλευσεν ετη εννεα. τουτον οἱ της τροφου αυτου υἱοι τεσσαρες επιβουλευσαντες απωλεσαν, ὡν ὁ πρεσβυτερος εβασιλευσεν ετη δεκαδυο. μεθ' οὑς Ασταρτος ὁ Δελαιασταρτου, ὁς, βιωσας ετη πεντηκοντα τεσσαρα, εβασιλευσεν ετη δωδεκα. μετα τουτον ὁ αδελφος αυτου Ασερυμος, βιωσας ετη τεσσαρα και πεντηκοντα, εβασιλευσεν ετη εννεα. οὑτος απωλετο ὑπο του ἀδελφου Φελητος, ὁς λαβων την βασιλειαν ηρξε μηνας οκτω, βιωσας ετη πεντηκοντα. τουτον ανειλεν Ειθωβαλος ὁ της Ασταρτης ἱερευς, ὁς, βασιλευσας ετη τριακοντα δυο, εβιωσεν ετη ἑξηκοντα οκτω. τουτον διεδεξατο Βαδεζωρος υἱος, ὁς,

Upon the death of Hiromus, Baleazarus his son succeeded to the kingdom; he lived forty-three years, and reigned seven: after him Abdastratus his son reigned nine years, having lived twenty-nine: against him the four sons of his nurse conspired, and slew him: of these the eldest reigned twelve years: after them Astartus, the son of Delæastartus, reigned twelve years, having lived fifty-four: after him his brother Aserumus reigned nine years, having lived fifty-four: he was slain by his brother Pheles, who governed the kingdom eight months, having lived fifty years: he was slain by a priest of Astarte, Ithobalus, who reigned thirty-two years, having lived sixty-eight: and he was succeeded by Badezorus his son, who reigned six years, having lived forty-five: his successor was Matgenus his son, who reigned nine years, having lived thirty-two: and he was succeeded by Phygmalion who reigned forty-seven years, having lived fifty-six: in the seventh year of his reign his sister βιωσας ετη τεσσαρακοντα πεντε, εβασιλευσεν ετη ἑξ. τουτου διαδοχος γεγονε Ματγηνος ὁ υἱος, ὁς, βιωσας ετη τριακοντα δυο, εβασιλευσεν ετη εννεα. τουτου διαδοχος γεγονε Φυγμαλιων, βιωσας δ' ετη πεντηκοντα ἑξ, εβασιλευσεν ετη τεσσαρακοντα ἑπτα. εν δε τῳ επ' αυτου ἑβδομῳ ετει ἡ αδελφη αυτου φυγουσα, εν τῃ Λιβυῃ πολιν ῳκοδομησε Καρχηδονα.

fled from him, and founded the city of Carthage in Libya.—*Joseph. contr. App.* lib. I. c. 18.

## OF THE INVASION OF SALMANASAR.

Και Ελουλαιος ονομα εβασιλευσεν ετη τριακοντα ἑξ. οὑτος, αποσταντων Κιτταιων, αναπλευσας, προσηγαγετο αυτους παλιν. επι τουτους πεμψας (Σαλμανασαρ) ὁ των Ασσυριων βασιλευς, επηλθε Φοινικην πολεμων ἁπασαν. ὁς τις σπεισαμενος ειρηνην, μετα παντων ανεχωρησεν οπισω. απεστη τε Τυριων Σιδων και Ακη και ἡ Παλαι Τυρος, και πολλαι αλλαι πολεις, αἱ τῳ των Ασσυριων ἑαυτας βασιλει παρεδοσαν. διο Τυριων ουχ ὑποταγεντων παλιν ὁ βασιλευς επ' αυτους ὑπεστρεψε, Φοινικων συμπληρωσαντων αυτῳ ναυς ἑξηκοντα, και επικωπους οκτακοσιους. αἱς επιπλευσαντες οἱ Τυριοι ναυσι

Elulæus reigned thirty-six years: and he fitted out a fleet against the Cittæans (Chittim or Cypriots) who had revolted, and reduced them to obedience. But Salmanasar, the king of the Assyrians, sent them assistance, and overran Phœnicia: and when he had made peace with the Phœnicians he returned with all his forces. And Sidon, and Ace (Acre), and Palætyrus, and many other cities revolted from the Tyrians, and put themselves under the protection of the king of Assyria. But as the Tyrians still refused to submit, the king made another expedition against them: and the Phœnicians furnished him with sixty ships and eighty gallies: and the Tyrians attacked him with twelve ships, and dispersed the hostile fleet, δεκαδυο, των νεων των αντιπαλων διασπαρεισων, λαμβανουσιν αιχμαλωτους ανδρας εις πεντακοσιους. επεταθη δη παντων εν Τυρῳ τιμη δια ταυτα. αναζευξας δ' ὁ των Ασσυριων βασιλευς καταστησε φυλακας επι του ποταμου και των ὑδραγωγιων, οἱ διακωλυσουσι Τυριους αρυσασθαι. και τουτο ετεσι πεντε γενομενον, εκαρτερησαν πινοντες εκ φρεατων ορυκτων.

and took prisoners to the amount of five hundred men: upon which account the Tyrians were held in great respect. But the king of Assyria stationed guards upon the river, and aqueducts, to prevent the Tyrians from drawing water: and this continued five years, during all which time they were obliged to drink from wells which they dug.—*Joseph. Antiq. Jud.* lib. IX. c. 14.

# THE TYRIAN ANNALS.

---

## OF THE KINGS AND JUDGES FROM NEBUCHADNEZZAR TO CYRUS.

ΕΠΙ Ειθωβαλου του βασιλεως επολιορκησε Ναβουχοδονοσορος την Τυρον επ' ετη δεκατρια μετα τουτον εβασιλευσε Βααλ ετη δεκα. μετα τουτον δικασται κατεσταθησαν και εδικασαν· Εκνιβαλος Βασληχου μηνας δυο, Χελβης Αβδαιου μηνας δεκα, Αββαρος αρχιερευς μηνας τρεις, Μυτγονος και Γεραστρατος του Αβδηλεμου δικασται ετη ἑξ, ὧν μεταξυ εβασιλευσε Βαλατορος ενιαυτον ἑνα· τουτου τελευτησαντος, αποστειλαντες μετεπεμψαντο Μερβαλον εκ της Βαβυλωνος, και εβασιλευσεν ετη τεσσαρα. τουτου τελευτησαντος, μετεπεμψαντο τον αδελφον αυτου Ειρωμον, ὁς εβασιλευσεν ετη εικοσιν. επι τουτου Κυρος Περσων εδυναστευσεν.

IN the reign of Ithobalus, Nabuchodonosorus besieged Tyre for thirteen years. After him reigned Baal ten years. After him Judges were appointed who judged the people: Ecnibalus, the son of Baslachus, two months: Chelbes, the son of Abdæus, ten months: Abbarus, the high-priest, three months: Mytgonus and Gerastratus the son of Abdelemus, six years: after them Balatorus reigned one year. After his death they sent to fetch Merbalus from Babylon: and he reigned four years: and when he died they sent for Hiromus, his brother, who reigned 20 years. In his time Cyrus was king of Persia.—*Joseph. contr. App.* lib. I. c. 21.

THE ORACLES

OF

# ZOROASTER.

THE ORACLES

OF

# ZOROASTER.

O

# ΤΑ ΤΟΥ ΖΩΡΟΑΣΤΡΟΥ ΛΟΓΙΑ.

---

## ΜΟΝΑΣ ΔΥΑΣ ΚΑΙ ΤΡΙΑΣ.

. . . . . . ʽΟΠΟΥ πατρικη μονας εστι.
Ταναη εστι μονας . . . . . ἡ δυο γεννᾳ
Δυας γαρ παρα τῳ δε καθηται, και νοεραις αστραπτει τομαις
Και το κυβερναν τα παντα, και ταττειν ἑκαστον ου ταχθεν.
Παντι γαρ εν κοσμῳ λαμπει τριας, ἡς μονας
αρχει.
Αρχη πασης τμησεως ἡ δε ἡ ταξις.
Εις τρια γαρ νους ειπε πατρος τεμνεσθαι ἁπαντα,
Οὗ το θελειν κατενευσε, και ηδη παντα ετετμητο
Εις τρια γαρ ειπε νους πατρος αϊδιου,
Νῳ παντα κυβερνων.
Και εφανησαν εν αυτῃ ἡ τ᾽ αρετη, και ἡ σοφια.
Και ἡ πολυφρων ατρεκεια.
Τῃ τῃδε ρεει τριαδος δεμας προ της ουσης,
Ου πρωτης, αλλ᾽ οὗ τα μετρειται.
Αρχαις γαρ τρισι ταις δε λαβοις δουλευειν ἁπαντα.
. . . . ʽΙερος πρωτος δρομος, εν δ᾽ αρα μεσσῳ.
Ηεριος, τριτος αλλος, ὃς εν πυρι την χθονα θαλπει.
Και πηγη πηγων, και πηγων . . . . ἁπασων.
Μητρα συνεχουσα τα παντα.
Ενθεν αρδην θρωσκει γενεσις πολυποικιλου ὑλης.

# THE ORACLES OF ZOROASTER.

## MONAD, DUAD, AND TRIAD.

. . . . . Where the paternal Monad is.
The Monad is enlarged, and generates two,
For the Duad sits by him, and glitters with intellectual Sections
Both to govern all things, and to order every thing not ordered.
For in the whole world shineth the Triad, over which the Monad rules.
This order is the beginning of all section.
For the mind of the Father said, that all things be cut into three:
Whose will assented, and then all things were divided.
For the mind of the Eternal Father said all things into three,
Governing all things by the mind.
And there appeared in it (the Triad) virtue, and wisdom,
And multiscient verity.
This way floweth the shape of the Triad, being pre-existent.
Not the first (Essence) but where they are measured.
For thou must conceive that all things serve these three principles.
The first is the sacred course . . . . but in the middle
Air, the third the other which cherisheth the earth in fire.
The fountain of fountains and . . . . of all fountains.
The matrix containing all things.
Thence abundantly springs forth the generation of multifarious matter.

Ενθεν συρομενος πρηστηρ αμυδροιο πυρος ανθος,
Κοσμων ενθρωσκων κοιλωμασι. Παντα γαρ ενθεν
Αρχεται εις το κατω τεινειν ακτινας αγητας.

## ΠΑΤΗΡ ΚΑΙ ΝΟΥΣ.

Ἑαυτον ὁ πατηρ ἡρπασεν ουδ᾽ εν ἑῃ
Δυναμει νοερᾳ κλεισας ιδιον πυρ.
Ου γαρ απο πατρικης αρχης ατελες τι τροχαζει.
Παντα γαρ εξετελεσε πατηρ,
Και νῳ παρεδωκε δευτερῳ,
Ὁν πρωτον κληιζεται παν γενος ανδρων.
Πατρογενες φαος, πολυ γαρ μονος
Εκ πατρος αλκης δρεψαμενος νοου ανθος.
Εργα νοησας, γαρ πατρικος νοος αυτογενεθλος,
Πασιν ενεσπειρε δεσμον περιβριθη ερωτος.
Οφρα τα παντα μενῃ, χρονον εις απεραντον ερωντα.
Μητε πεσοι τα πατρος νοερως ὑφασμενα
        φεγγει.
Ὡς εν ερωτι μενῃ κοσμου στοιχεια μενοντα.
Εχει τῳ νοειν πατρικον νουν ενδιδοναι
Πασαις πηγαις τε και αρχαις.
Εστι γαρ περας του πατρικου βαθου, και πηγη των
        νοερων.
Μη δε προηλθεν, αλλ᾽ εμενεν εν τῳ πατρικῳ βαθῳ,
Και εν τῳ αδυτῳ, κατα την θεοθρεμμονα σιγην.
Ου γαρ εις ὑλην, πυρ επεκεινα το πρωτον
Εην δυναμιν κατακλειει εργοις, αλλα νῳ.
Συμβολα γαρ πατρικος νοος εσπειρε κατα κοσμον.
Ὁς τα νοητα νοει και αφραστα καλληΐται.
Ὁλοφυης μερισμος, και αμεριστος.
Νῳ μεν κατεχει τα νοητα, αισθησιν δ᾽ επαγει
        κοσμοις.
Νῳ μεν κατεχει τα νοητα, ψυχην δ᾽ επαγει κοσμοις.

Thence extracted a Prester the flower of glowing fire,
Flashing into the cavities of the World: For all things from thence
Begin to extend downward their admirable beams.

### THE FATHER AND MIND.

The Father hath snatched away himself; neither
Hath he shut up his own fire in his intellectual power.
For nothing unfinished proceedeth from the Father's rule.
For the Father perfected all things,
And delivered them over to the second mind,
Which the whole race of men call the first.
Light begotten of the Father, for he alone
Having cropt the flower of the Mind from the Father's vigor.
For the paternal self-begotten Mind understanding (his) work,
Sowed in all the fiery bond of Love,
That all things might continue loving for ever.
Neither those things which are intellectually context in the Light of the Father in all things.
That being the Elements of the World they might persist in Love.
For by understanding he hath the power to instil the paternal mind
Into all fountains and beginnings.
For it is the bound of the Paternal depth and the fountain of the Intellectuals.
Neither went he forth, but abode in the Paternal depth,
And in the Adytum according to divinely-nourished Silence.
For the fire once above, shutteth not his power
Into matter by Actions, but by the Mind.
For the Paternal Mind hath sowed symbols through the world.
Which understandeth intelligibles and beautifieth ineffables.
Wholly division and indivisible.
By mind he contains the Intelligibles, but introduceth sense into the Worlds.
By mind he contains the Intelligibles, but introduceth Soul into the Worlds.

## ΝΟΥΣ, ΝΟΗΤΑ, ΚΑΙ ΝΟΕΡΑ.

Και του ἑνος νου του νοητου.

Ου γαρ ανευ νοος εστι νοητου· ου χωρις ὑπαρχει.

Τα μεν εστι νοερα και νοητα, ὁσα νοουντα
νοειται.

Τροφη δε τῳ νοουντι το νοητον.

Μανθανε το νοητον, επει νοου εξω ὑπαρχει.

Και του νου, ὁς τον εμπυριον κοσμον αγει.

Νου γαρ νους εστιν ὁ κοσμου τεχνιτης πυριου.

Οἱ τον ὑπερκοσμιον πατρικον βυθον ιστε νοουντες.

Ἡ νοητη πασης τμησεως αγει.

Εστι γαρ τι νοητον, ὁ χρη σε νοειν νοου
ανθει.

Ἡ γαρ επεγκλινης, ὡς αν νουν, κακεινο νοησῃς,
Ὡς τι νοων, ου κεινον
νοησεις

Εστι γαρ αλκης αμφιφαους δυναμις,
Νοεραις στραπτουσα τομαισι, ου δη χρη
Σφοδροτητι νοειν το νοητον εκεινο.
Αλλα νοου ταναου ταναῃ φλογι
Παντα μετρουσῃ, πλην το νοητον εκεινο.
Χρεω δη τουτο νοησαι· η γαρ επεγκλινης
Σον νουν, κακεινο νοησεις ουκ αντενας.
Αλλ' ἁγνον επιστρεφον ομμα,
Φεροντα σης ψυχης τειναι κενεον νοον
Εις το νοητον, οφρα μαθῃς το νοητον·
Επει εξω νοου ὑπαρχει.

Τον δε νοει πας νους θεον, ου γαρ
ανευ
Νους εστι νοητου, και το νοητον ου νου χωρις ὑπαρχει.

Τοις δε πυρος νοερου νοεροις πρηστηρσιν ἁπαντα
Εικαθε δουλευοντα, πατρος πειθηνιδι βουλῃ.

## MIND, INTELLIGIBLES, AND INTELLECTUALS.

And of the one Mind, the Intelligible (Mind).
For the Mind is not without the Intelligible; it exists not without it.
These are Intellectuals and Intelligibles which being understood understand.
For the Intelligible is the aliment of the Intelligent.
Learn the Intelligible, since it exists beyond the Mind.
And of the Mind which moves the empyreal heaven.
For the Framer of the fiery world is the Mind of the Mind.
You who know certainly the supermundane paternal depth.
The Intelligible is predominant over all section.
There is something Intelligible which it behoves thee to understand with the flower of the Mind.
For if thou inclinest thy mind, thou shalt understand this also.
Yet understanding something (of it) thou shalt not understand this wholly;
For it is a power of circumlucid strength,
Glittering with intellectual sections (rays): but it behoves not
To consider this Intelligible with vehemence of Intellection,
But with the ample flame of the ample Mind
Which measureth all things, except this Intelligible:
But it behoves to understand this; for if thou inclinest
Thy mind thou shalt understand this also, not fixedly
But having a pure turning eye (thou must)
Extend the empty mind of thy soul
Towards the Intelligible; that thou mayest learn the Intelligible;
For it exists beyond the mind.
But every mind understands this God; for the Mind is not
Without the Intelligible, neither is the Intelligible without the Mind.
To the Intellectual Presters of the intellectual fire all things
By yielding are subservient to the persuasive counsel of the Father,

Και τα νοειν, αει τε μενειν αοκνῳ στροφαλιγγι.
Πηγας τε και αρχας, δινειν, αει τε μενειν αοκνῳ
    στροφαλιγγι.
Αλλα δ' ουνομα σεμνον ακοιμητῳ
    στροφαλιγγι
Κοσμοις ενθρωσκων, κραιπνην δια πατρος ενιπην.
Ὑπο δυο νοων ἡ ζωογονος πηγη περιεχεται
    ψυχων.
Και ὁ ποιητης, ὁς αυτουργων τεκτηνατο τον κοσμον.
Ὁς εκ νοου εκθορε πρωτος.
Εσσαμενος πυρι πυρ, συνδεσμων οφρα κεραση
Πηγαιους κρατηρας, ἑου πυρος ανθος επισχων.
Νοεραις αστραπτει τομαις, ερωτος δ'ενεπλησε τα
    παντα.
Τα ατυπωτα τυπουσθαι.
Σμηνεσσιν εοικυιαι φερονται, ῥηγνυμεναι
Κοσμου περι σωμασι.
Ἁ νους λεγει, τῳ νοειν δη που λεγει.
Ἡ μεν γαρ δυναμις συν εκεινοις, νους δ' απ' εκεινου.

## ΙΥΝΓΕΣ, ΙΔΕΑΙ ΑΡΚΑΙ.

Πολλαι μεν αἱδε επεμβαινουσι φαεινοις κοσμοις.
Ενθρωσκουσαι, και εν αἱς ακροτητες εασι τρεις,
Ὑποκειται αυταις αρχηις αυλων.
Αρχας, αἱ πατρος εργα νοησασαι
    νοητα
Αισθητοις εργοις, και σωμασιν αμφεκαλυψεν.
Δια πορθμιοι ἑστωτες φαναι τῳ πατρι και τη ὑλη.
Και τα εμφανη μιμηματα των αφανων εργαζομενοι.
Και τ' αφανη εις την εμφανη κοσμοποιΐαν εγγραφοντες.
Νους πατρος ερῤοιζησε, νοησας ακμαδι
    βουλη
Παμμορφους ιδεας. πηγης δ' απο μιας αποπτασαι
Εξεθορον. πατροθεν γαρ εην βουλη τε τελος τε

And to understand, and always to remain in a restless whirling.
Fountains and principles, to turn, and always to remain in a restless whirling.
By insinuating into Worlds the venerable name in a sleepless whirling
By reason of the terrible menace of the Father.
Under two Minds the life-generating fountain of the Souls is contained.
And the Maker who, self-operating, framed the World.
Who sprung first out of the Mind.
Clothing fire with fire, binding them together to mingle
The fountainous craters, preserving the flower of his own fire.
He glittereth with Intellectual sections, and filleth all things with love.
That things unfashioned may be fashioned.
Like swarms they are carried, being broken
About the bodies of the world.
What the Mind speaks, it speaks by understanding.
Power is with them—mind is from her.

## IYNGES, IDEAS, AND PRINCIPLES.

These being many ascend into the lucid Worlds,
Springing into them, and in which are three tops.
Beneath them lies the chief of Immaterials.
Principles, which have understood the intelligible works of the Father,
Disclosed them in sensible works as in bodies:
Being (as it were) the ferrymen betwixt the Father and matter.
And producing manifest images of unmanifest things:
And inscribing the unmanifest in the manifest frame of the World.
The Mind of the Father made a jarring noise, understanding by vigorous counsel
Omniform Ideas: and flying out of one fountain
They sprung forth: for from the Father was the counsel and end

Δι' ὧν συναπτεται τῳ πατρι, αλλην κατ' αλλην
Ζωην, απο μεριζομενων οχετων.
Αλλ' εμερισθησαν, νοερῳ πυρι μοιρηθεισαι
Εις αλλας νοερας· κοσμῳ γαρ αναξ
πολυμορφῳ
Προυθηκεν νοερον τυπον αφθιτον, οὗ κατα κοσμον
Ιχνος επειγομενος μορφης καθ' ἁ κοσμος
εφανθη,
Παντοιαις ιδεαις κεχαρισμενος, ὧν μια πηγη,
Εξ ἧς ῥοιζουνται μεμερισμεναι αλλαι,
Απλατοι, ῥηγνυμεναι κοσμου περι σωμασι·
Αἱ περι κολπους σμερδαλεους, σμηνεσσιν εοικυιαι,
Φορεονται τραπουσαι περι δ' αμφι αλλυδις αλλη.
Εννοιαι νοεραι πηγης πατρικης απο
Πολυ δραττομεναι πυρος ανθος
Ακοιμητου χρονου, ακμη αρχεγονου ιδεας
Πρωτη πατρος εβλυσε· τας δ' αυτοθαλης πηγη.
Νοουμεναι ιϋγγες πατροθεν νοεουσι και αυται.
Βουλαις αφθεγκτοισι κινουμεναι ὡστε νοησαι.

## ἙΚΑΤΗ, ΣΥΝΟΧΕΙΣ, ΚΑΙ ΤΕΛΕΑΡΧΑΙ

Εξ αυτου γαρ παντες εκθρωσκουσι
Αμειλικτοι τε κεραυνοι, και πρηστηροδοχοι κολποι
Παμφεγγεος αλκης πατρογενους Ἑκατης.
Και ὑπεζωκος πυρος ανθος, ἡ δε κραταιον
Πνευμα πολων, πυριων επεκεινα.
Φρουρειν αυ πρηστηρσιν ἑοις ακροτητας εδωκεν.
Εγκερασας αλκης ιδιον μενος εν συνοχευσιν.
Ω πας εχει κοσμος νοερους ανοχηας απαμπεις.
Ὁτι εργατις, ὁτι εκδοτις εστι πυρος
ζωηφορου.
Ὁτι και το ζωογονον πληροι της Ἑκατης κολπον.
Και επιρῥει τοις συνοχευσιν αλκην ζωδοτον πυρος,
Μεγα δυναμενου.

By which they are connected with the Father by alternate
Life from several vehicles.
But they were divided, being by intellectual fire distributed
Into other Intellectuals: for the king did set before the multiform world
An intellectual incorruptible pattern: the print of whose form
He promoted through the world, according to which things the world appeared
Beautified with all kinds of Ideas, of which there is one fountain;
Out of which come rushing forth others undistributed,
Being broken about the bodies of the World;
Which through the vast recesses, like swarms,
Are carried round about every way.
Intellectual notions from the paternal fountain
Cropping the flower of Fire
In the point of sleepless time of this primigeneous Idea
The first self-budding fountain of the Father budded.
Intelligent Iynges do (themselves) also understand from the Father:
By unspeakable counsels being moved so as to understand.

## HECATE, SYNOCHES, AND TELETARCHS.

For out of him spring all
Implacable thunders, and the prester-receiving cavities
Of the entirely-lucid strength of Father-begotten Hecate.
And he who begirds (viz.) the flower of Fire and the strong
Spirit of the poles fiery above.
He gave to his presters that they should guard the tops.
Mingling the power of his own strength in the Synoches.
Oh how the world hath intellectual guides inflexible!
Because she is the operatrix, because she is the dispensatrix of fire-giving life.
Because also it fills the life-producing bosom of Hecate,
And instils in the Synoches the enlivening strength
Of potent fire.

Ἀλλα και φρουροι των εργων εισι του πατρος.
Αφομοιοι γαρ ἑαυτον, εκεινος επειγομενος
Τον τυπον περιβαλλεσθαι των ειδωλων.
Οἱ τελεταρχαι συνειληπται τοις συνοχευσι.
Τοις δε πυρος νοερου νοερους πρηστηρσιν
Ἁπαντα εικαθε δουλευοντα.
Αλλα και ὑλαιοις ὁσα δουλευει συνοχευσι.
Ἑσσαμενοι παντευχον αλκην φωτος κελαδοντος.
Αλκη τριγλωχι, νοον ψυχην τ' ὁπλισαντα
Παντοιαδος συνθημα βαλλειν φρενι.
Μηδ' επιφοιταν εμπυριοις σποραδην οχετοις,
Αλλα στιβαρηδον.
Οἱ δε τα ατομα, και αισθητα δημιουργουσι,
Και σωματοειδη, και κατατεταγμενα εις ὑλην.

## ΨΥΧΗ, ΦΥΣΙΣ.

Ὁτι ψυχη πυρ δυναμει πατρος ουσα φαεινον,
Αθανατος τε μενει, και ζωης δεσποτις εστι
Και ισχει κοσμου πολλα πληρωματα κολπων.
Νου γαρ μιμημα πελει, το δε τεχθεν εχει τι
σωματος.
Μιγνυμενων δ' οχετων, πυρος αφθιτου εργα
τελουσα.
Μετα δε πατρικας διανοιας ψυχη εγω, ναιω
Θερμη, ψυχουσα τα παντα, κατεθετο γαρ
Νουν μεν ενι ψυχη, ψυχην δ' ενι σωματι αργῳ
Ἡμεων εγκατεθηκε πατηρ ανδρων τε θεων τε.
Αρδην εμψυχουσα φαος, πυρ, αιθερα, κοσμους.
Συνιστανται γαρ τα φυσικα εργα τῳ νοερῳ φεγγει
Του πατρος· Ψυχη γαρ κοσμησασα τον μεγαν
Ουρανον, και κοσμουσα μετα του πατρος.
Κερατα δε και αυτης εστηρικται αυω.
Νωτοις δ' αμφι θεας φυσις απλετος
ηωρηται.

But they are guardians of the works of the Father.
For he assimilates himself, professing
To be clothed with the print of the images.
The Teletarchs are comprehended with the Synoches.
To those intellectual presters of intellectual fire
All things are subservient.
But as many as serve the material Synoches
Having put on the completely-armed vigour of resounding light,
With triple strength fortifying the soul and the mind
To put into the mind the symbol of variety.
And not to walk dispersedly on the empyreal channels
But firmly.
These frame indivisibles and sensibles,
And corporiforms and things destined to matter.

### SOUL, NATURE.

The Soul being a bright fire, by the power of the Father,
Remains immortal and is mistress of life:
And possesseth many complexions of the cavities of the world:
For it is an imitation of the Mind; but that which is born hath something of the body.
The channels being intermixed she performs the part of incorruptible fire.
Next the paternal conception, I, the soul dwell;
Warmth heating all things, for he did put
The mind in the soul, the soul in the dull body.
Of us the father of gods and men interposed.
Abundantly animating light, fire, ether, worlds.
For natural works co-exist with the intellectual light
Of the Father. For the soul which adorned the great
Heaven, and adorning with the Father,
But her horns are fixed above:
But about the shoulders of the Goddess Immense Nature is exalted.

Αρχει δ' αυ φυσις ακαματη κοσμων τε και εργων·
Ουρανος οφρα θεει δρομον αΐδιον κατασυρων·
Και ταχυς ἠελιος περι κεντρον, ὁπως εθας ελθη.
Μη φυσεως εμβλεψεις εἱμαρμενον ουνομα τησδε.

## ΚΟΣΜΟΣ.

Ὁ ποιητης ὁς αυτουργων τεκταινετο τον κοσμον.
Και τις πυρος ογκος εην ἑτερος· τα δε παντα
Αυτουργων, ἱνα σωμα το κοσμικον εκτολυπευθη,
Κοσμος ἱν' εκδηλος, και μη φαινηται ὑμενωδης.
Τον ὁλον κοσμον εκ πυρος, και ὑδατος, και γης,
Και παντοτροφου αιθερος.
Τ' αρρητα, και τα ῥητα συνθηματα του κοσμου.
Αλλη κατ' αλλην ζωνην, απο μεριζομενων οχετων.
Ανωθεν διηκοντος επι το κατ' αντικρυ
Δια του κεντρου της γης, και πεμπτον μεσον, αλλον
Περιοχη, ενθα κατεισι μεχρι ὑλαιων οχετων.
Ζωηφορον πυρ.
Κεντρω επι ῥοιζων ἑαυτου φωτος κελαδοντος
Πηγαιων αλλων, ὁς τους εμπυριους κοσμους αγει.
Κεντρον αφ' οὑ πασαι μεχρις αν τυχοι ισαι εασι.
Συμβολα γαρ πατρικος νους εσπειρε κατα κοσμον.
Μεσον των πατερων Ἑκατης κεντρον φερεσθαι.
Νου γαρ μιμημα πελει· το δε τεχθεν εχει τι
σωματος.

## ΟΥΡΑΝΟΣ.

Ἑπτα γαρ εξωγκωσε πατηρ στερεωματα κοσμων·
Τον ουρανον κυρτω σχηματι περικλεισας.
Πηξε δε πολυν ὁμιλον αστερων απλανων
Ζωων και πλανωμενων [illegible] ἑπταδα.
Γην δ' εν μεσσω πυρος, ὑδωρ δ' εν γαιης κολποις,

Again indefatigable Nature commands the worlds and works;
That Heaven drawing an eternal course might run,
And the swift sun might come about the centre as he useth.
Look not into the fatal name of this Nature.

## THE WORLD.

The Maker who operating by himself framed the World.
And there was another bulk of fire, self-operating
All things, that the body of the World might be perfected.
That the World might be manifest, and not seem membranous.
The whole World of fire, and water, and earth,
And all-nourishing ether.
The inexpressible and expressible watchwords of the World.
One life with another, from the distributed channels.
Passing from above through the opposite part
Through the centre of the Earth; and another fifth the middle,
Another fiery channel, where it descends to the material channels.
Life-bringing fire.
Stirring himself up with the goad of resounding light.
Another fountainous, which guides the empyreal World.
The centre from which all (lines) which way soever are equal.
For the paternal Mind sowed symbols through the World
For the centre of every one is carried betwixt the Fathers.
For it is an imitation of the Mind, but that which is born hath
something of the Body.

## HEAVEN.

For the Father congregated seven firmaments of the World,
Circumscribing Heaven in a round figure.
And fixed a great company of inerratic stars.
And he constituted a septennary of erratic animals.
Placing earth in the middle, and water in the middle of the earth.

Πυρα δ' αναθεν τουτων.
Πηξε δε και πολυν όμιλον αστερων απλανων.
Μη τασει επιπονῳ πονηρῃ
Πηξῃ δε πλανην ουκ εχουσῃ φερεσθαι.
Επηξε δε και πολυν όμιλον αστερων απλανων.
Το πυρ προς το πυρ αναγκασας.
Πηξῃ πλανην ουκ εχουσῃ φερεσθαι.
Ἑξ αυτους ὑπεστησεν, ἑβδομον ἡλιου.
Μεσεμβολησας πυρ.
Το ατακτον αυτων ευτακτοις αναρτημασιν ζωννυς.
Τικτει γαρ ἡ ῥεα, ἡελιον τε μεγαν και λαμπραν σεληνην.
Αιθηρ, ἡλιε, πνευμα σεληνης, αερος αγοι,
Ἡλιακων τε κυκλων, και μηναιων καναχισμων.
Κολπων τε ηεριων.
Αιθρης μελος, ἡελιου τε, και μηνης οχετων, ἠ τε
ηερος.
Και πλατυς αηρ, μηναιος τε δρομος. και πολος ἡελιοιο.
Συλλεγει αυτο, λαμβανουσα αιθρης μελος,
Ἡελιου τε, σεληνης τε, και ὁσα ηερι
συνεχονται.
Πυρ πυρος εξοχετευμα, και πυρος ταμιας.
Χαιται γαρ ες οξυ πεφρικοτι φωτι βλεπονται,
Ενθα Κρονος.
Ἡελιος παρεδρος επισκοπεων πολον αγνον.
Αιθεριος τε δρομος και μηνης απλετος ὁρμη,
Ηερια τε ῥοαι.
Ἡελιον τε [illegible], και λαμπραν σεληνην.

## ΧΡΟΝΟΣ.

Θεον εγκοσμιον, αιωνιον, απεραντον.
Νεον και πρεσβυτην, ἑλικοειδη.
Και τυγχανει αλλον ὁς τον εμπυριον κοσμον αγει.

The air above these.
He fixed a great company of inerratic stars,
To be carried not by laborious and troublesome tension,
But by a settlement which hath no error.
He fixed a great company of inerratic stars,
Forcing fire to fire.
To be carried by a settlement which hath no error.
He constituted them six, casting into the midst
The seventh fire of the sun.
Suspending their disorder in well-ordered zones.
For the goddess brings forth the great sun and the bright moon.
Oh ether, sun, spirit of the moon, guides of the air,
And of the solar circles, and of the lunar clashings
And of the aerial recesses!
The melody of the ether, and of the passages of the sun and moon, and of the air.
And the wide air, and the lunar course, and the pole of the sun,
It collects it, receiving the melody of the ether,
And of the sun, and of the moon, and of all things that are contained in the air.
Fire the derivation of fire, and the dispenser of fire.
His hair pointed is seen by his native light,
Hence Cronus.
The sun assessor beholding the pure pole
And the ethereal course and the vast motion of the moon,
And the aerial fluxions.
And the great sun, and the bright moon.

## TIME.

The mundane god eternal, infinite.
Young and old, and of a spiral form,
And another fountainous who guides the empyreal heaven.

## ΨΥΧΗ, ΣΩΜΑ, ΑΝΘΡΩΠΟΣ.

Χρη σε σπευδειν προς το φαος και πατρος αυγας,
Ενθεν επεμφθη σοι ψυχη, πολυν ἑσσαμενη νουν.
Ταυτα πατηρ ενοησε, βροτος δ' οἱ εψυχωτο.
Συμβολα γαρ πατρικος νοος εσπειρε ταις ψυχαις,
Ερωτι βαθει αναπλησας την ψυχην.
Κατεθετο γαρ νουν εν ψυχη, εν σωματι δε
Ὑμεας εγκατεθηκε πατηρ ανδρων τε θεων τε.
Ασωματα μεν εστι τα θεια παντα.
Σωματα δ' εν αυτοις ὑμων ἑνεκεν ενδεδεται.
Μη δυναμενους κατασχειν ασωματους των σωματων.
Δια την σωματικην, εις ἡν ενεκεντρισθητε, φυσιν.
Εν δε θεῳ κεινται πυρσους ἑλκουσαι ακμαιους.
Εκ πατροθεν κατιοντες, αφ' ὡν ψυχη κατιοντων
Εμπυριων δρεπεται καρπων, ψυχοτροφον ανθος.
Διο και νοησασι τα εργα του πατρος
Μοιρης εἱμαρμενης το πτερον φευγουσιν αναιδες.
Καν γαρ τηνδε ψυχην ιδης αποκαταστασαν,
Αλλ' αλλην ενιησι πατηρ, εναριθμιον ειναι.
Ἡ μαλα δε κειναι γε μακαρταται εξοχα πασεων
Ψυχαων, ποτι γαιαν απ' ουρανοθεν προχεονται.
Κειναι ολβιαι τε, και ου φατα νειματα εχουσαι.
Ὁσσαι απ' αιγληεντος, αναξ, σεθεν, η δε και αυτου
Εκ Διος εξεγενοντο, μιτου κρατερης ὑπ' αναγκης.
Ἡγεισθω ψυχης βαθος αμβροτον, ομματα δ'
αρδην
Παντα εκπετασον ανω.
Μητε κατω νευσεις εις τον μελαναυγεα κοσμον.
Ὡ βαθος αιεν απιστος ὑπεστρωται τε, και Ἁδης
Αμφινεφης, ῥυπων, ειδωλοχαρης, ανοητος,
Κρημνωδης, σκολιος, πωρον βαθος αιεν ἑλισσων,
Αει νυμφευων αφανες δεμας, αργον, απνευμον.

## SOUL, BODY, MAN.

It behoves thee to hasten to the light, and the beams of the Father,
From whence was sent to thee a Soul clothed with much Mind.
These things the Father conceived, and so the mortal was animated.
For the paternal Mind sowed symbols in Souls,
Replenishing the Soul with profound love.
For the Father of Gods and Men placed the Mind in the Soul,
And in the Body he established you.
For all divine things are incorporeal.
But bodies are bound in them for your sakes:
Incorporeals not being able to contain the bodies
By reason of the corporeal nature in which you are concentrated.
And they are in God, attracting strong flames.
Descending from the Father, from which descending the Soul
Crops of empyreal fruits the soul-nourishing flower.
And therefore conceiving the works of the Father
They avoid the audacious wing of fatal destiny.
And though you see this soul manumitted,
Yet the Father sends another to make up the number.
Certainly these are superlatively blessed above all
Souls; they are sent forth from heaven to earth.
And those rich souls, which have inexpressible fates,
As many of them (O king) as proceed from shining thee,
Or from Jove himself, under the strong power of his thread,
Let the immortal depth of thy Soul be predominant; but thine eyes
Extend upwards.
Stoop not down to the dark world.
Beneath which continually lies a faithless depth and Hades
Dark all over, squalid, delighting in images unintelligible,
Precipitous, craggy, always involving a dark abyss,
Always espousing an opacous, idle, breathless body.

Και ὁ μισυφανης κοσμος, και τα σκολια ῥειθρα
Ὑφ' ὧν πολλοι κατασειρονται.
Ζητησον παραδεισον.
Διζεο συ ψυχης οχετον, ὁθεν, η τινι ταξει
Σωματι τιθυσας, επι ταξιν αφ' ἡς
ερρυης
Αυθις αναστησεις, ἱερῳ λογῳ εργον ἑνωσας.
Μητε κατω νευσεις, κρημνος κατα γης ὑποκειται.
Ἑπταπορου συρων κατα βαθμιδος· ἡν
ὑπο
Δεινης αναγκης θρονος εστι.
Μη συ αυξανε την εἱμαρμενην.
Ψυχη ἡ μεροπων θεον αγξει πως εις ἑαυτην.
Ουδεν θνητον εχουσα, ὁλη θεοθεν μεμεθευσται.
Ἁρμονιαν αυχει γαρ, ὑφ' ᾗ πελε σωμα βροτειον.
Εκτεινας πυριον νουν εργον επ' ευσεβιης,
Ῥευστον και σωμα σαωσεις.
Εστι και ειδωλῳ μερις εις τοπον αμφιφαοντα.
Παντοθεν ατλαστῳ ψυχη πυρος ἡνια τεινον.
Ἡ περιθαλπης εννοια πρωτιστην εχει ταξιν.
Τῳ πυρι γαρ βροτος εμπελασας θεοθεν φαος ἑξει.
Δηθυνοντι γαρ βροτῳ κρεπνοι μακαρες τελεθουσι.
Αἱ ποιναι μεροπων αγκτειραι.
Και τα κακης ὑλης βλαστηματα χρηστα, και εσθλα.
Ελπις τρεφετω σε πυριοχος αγγελικῳ ενι χωρῳ.
Αλλ' ουκ εισδεχεται κεινης το θελειν πατρικος νους.
Μεχρις αν εξελθη ληθης, και ῥημα λαλησῃ
Μνημην εισθεμενη πατρικου συνθηματος αγνου.
Τοις δε διδακτον φαους εδωκε γνωρισμα λαβεσθαι.
Τους δε ὑπνωοντας ἑης ενεκαρπισεν αλκης.
Μη πνευμα μολυνης μητε βαθυνης το επιπεδον.
Μητε το της ὑλης σκυβαλον κρημνῳ καταλειψεις.
Μη εξαξης, ἱνα μη εξιουσα εχη τι.
Βιῃ ὁτι σωμα λιποντων ψυχαι καθαρωταται.
Ψυχης εξωστηρες αναπνοοι, ευλυτοι
εισι.

And the light-hating world, and the winding currents
By which many things are swallowed up.
Seek Paradise.
Seek thou the way of the Soul, whence, and by what order
Having served the body, to the same place from which thou didst flow,
Thou mayest rise up again, joining action to sacred speech.
Stoop not down, for a precipice lies below the Earth,
Drawing through the ladder which hath seven steps; beneath which
Is the throne of necessity.
Enlarge not thy destiny.
The Soul of men will in a manner clasp God to herself.
Having nothing mortal she is wholly inebriated from God.
For she boasts harmony, in which the mortal body exists.
If thou extend the fiery mind to the work of piety,
Thou shalt preserve the fluxible body.
There is a room for the image also in the circumlucid place.
Every way to the unfashioned soul stretch the reins of fire.
The fire-glowing cogitation hath the first rank.
For the mortal approaching to the fire shall have light from God.
For to the slow mortal the Gods are swift.
The furies are stranglers of men.
The bourgeons even of ill matter are profitable and good.
Let fiery hope nourish thee in the angelic region,
But the paternal Mind accepts not her will,
Until she go out of oblivion and pronounce a word
Inserting the remembrance of the pure paternal symbol.
To these he gave the docile character of life to be comprehended.
Those that were asleep he made fruitful by his own strength.
Defile not the spirit nor deepen a superficies.
Leave not the dross of matter on a precipice.
Bring her not forth, lest going forth she have something.
The souls of those who quit the body violently are most pure.
The ungirders of the soul which give her breathing are easy to be loosed.

Λαιησ' εν λαγοσιν 'Εκατης αρετης πελε πηγη'
Ενδον ὁλη μιμνουσα, το παρθενον ου προϊεισα.
Ω τολμηροτατης φυσεως, ανθρωπε, τεχνασμα,
Μη τα πελωρια μετρα γαιης ὑπο σην φρενα βαλλου,
Ου γαρ αληθειης φυτον ενι χθονι.
Μητε μετρει μετρα ἠελιου κανονας συναθροισας,
Αϊδιῳ βουλῃ φερεται, ουχ ἑνεκα σοιο.
Μηναιον μεν δρομημα, και αστεριον
προπορευμα
Μηνης ῥοιζον εασον, αει τρεχει εργῳ αναγκης.
Αστεριον προπορευμα, σεθεν χαριν ουκ ελοχευθη.
Αιθεριος ορνιθων ταρσος πλατυς ου ποτ' αληθης,
Ου θυσιων σπλαγχνων τε τομαι· ταδ' αθυρματα παντα,
Εμποριχης απατης στηριγματα· φευγε συ ταυτα
Μελλων ευσεβιης ἱερον παραδεισον ανοιγειν.
Ενθ' αρετη, σοφια τε, και ευνομια συναγονται.
Σον γαρ αγγειον θηρες χθονος οικησουσι.
Αυτους δε χθων κατωρικται ες τεκνα μεχρις.

ΔΑΙΜΟΝΕΣ, ΤΕΛΕΤΑΙ.

Ἡ φυσις πειθει ειναι τους δαιμονας αγνους.
Και τα κακης ὑλης βλαστηματα χρηστα, και εσθλα.
Αλλα ταυτα εν αβατοις σηκοις διανοιας ανελιττω.
Πυρ ικελον σκιρτηδον επ' ηερος οιδμα τιταινων,
Η και πυρ ατυπωτον, ὁθεν φωνην προθεουσαν,
Η φως πλουσιον, αμφιγεινη ῥοιζουν, ελιχθεν·
Αλλα και ἱππον ιδειν φωτος πλεον αστραπτοντα,
Η και παιδα τεοις νωτοις εποχουμενον ἱππου,
Εμπυρον η χρυσῳ πεπυκασμενον, η παλιγυμνον,
Η και τοξευοντα, και εστωτα επι νωτοις,
Πολλακις ην λεξης μοι, αθρησης παντα
λεοντα,
Ουτε γαρ ουρανιος κυρτος τοτε φαινεται ογκος.
Αστερες ου λαμπουσι, το μηνης φως κεκαλυπται,

In the side of sinister Hecate there is a fountain of virtue;
Which remains entire within, not omitting her virginity.
Oh man, the machine of boldest nature!
Subject not to thy mind the vast measures of the earth,
For the plant of truth is not upon earth.
Nor measure the measures of the sun, gathering together canons,
He is moved by the eternal will of the Father not for thy sake.
Let alone the swift course of the moon and the progression of the stars,
For she runs always by the impulse of necessity.
And the progression of the stars was not brought forth for thy sake.
The ethereal wide flight of birds is not veracious,
And the dissections of entrails of victims; all these are toys,
The supports of gainful cheats; fly thou these
If thou intendest to open the sacred paradise of piety;
Where virtue, wisdom, and equity are assembled.
For thy vessel the beasts of the earth shall inhabit,
And the earth bewails them even to their children.

## DEMONS, RITES.

Nature persuades that there are pure Demons.
The bourgeons even of ill matter are profitable and good.
But these things I revolve in the recluse temples of my mind.
Extending the like fire sparklingly into the spacious air,
Or fire unfigured whence a voice issuing forth,
Or light abundant; whizzing and winding about the earth.
But also to see a horse more glittering than light,
Or a boy on thy shoulders riding on a horse,
Fiery or adorned with gold, or divested,
Or shooting, or standing on thy shoulders,
If thou speakest often to me thou shalt see absolutely that which is spoken,
For then neither appears the celestial concave bulk,
Nor do the stars shine, the light of the moon is covered,

Χθων ουκ ἑστηκε, βλεπεται τε παντα κεραυνοις.
Μη φυσεως καλεσῃς αυτοπτρον αγαλμα,
Ου γαρ χρη κεινους σε βλεπειν πριν σωμα τελεσθῃ·
Ὁτε τας ψυχας θελγοντες αει των τελετων
απαγουσι.
Εκ δ' αρα κολπων γαιης θρωσκουσι χθονιοι κυνες,
Ου ποτ' αληθες σωμα βροτῳ ανδρι δεικνυντες,
Ενεργει περι τον Ἑκατικον στροφαλον.
Ονοματα βαρβαρα μηποτ' αλλαξῃς,
Εισι γαρ ονοματα παρ' ἑκαστοις θεοσδοτα
Δυναμιν εν τελεταις αῤῥητον εχοντα.
Ἡνικα βλεψῃς μορφης ατερ ευίερον πυρ,
Λαμπομενον σκιρτηδον ὁλου κατα βενθεα κοσμου,
Κλυθι πυρος φωνην.

## ΘΕΟΣ.

Ὁ δε θεος εστι κεφαλην εχων ἱερακος· οὑτος εστιν ὁ πρωτος αφθαρτος, αΐδιος, αγεννητος, αμερης, ανομοιοτατος, ἡνιοχος παντος καλου, αδωροδοκητος, αγαθων αγαθωτατος, φρονιμων φρονιμωτατος. εστι δε και πατηρ ευνομιας και δικαιοσυνης, αυτοδιδακτος, φυσικος, και τελειος, και σοφος, και ἱερου φυσικου μονος εὑρετης.

The Earth stands not still, but all things appear in thunders.
Invoke not the self-conspicuous image of Nature,
For thou must not behold these before thy body is initiated:
When soothing souls they always seduce them from these mysteries.
Certainly out of the cavities of the Earth spring terrestrial dogs,
Which show no true sign to mortal man.
Labour about the Hecatick Strophalus.
Never change barbarous names,
For there are names in every nation given from God,
Which have an unspeakable power in Rites.
When thou seest a sacred fire without form,
Shining flashingly through the depths of the World,
Hear the voice of fire.

## GOD.

But God is he that has the head of a hawk. He is the first indestructible, eternal, unbegotten, indivisible, dissimilar; the dispenser of all good; incorruptible; the best of the good, the wisest of the wise: he is the father of equity and justice, self-taught, physical, and perfect, and wise, and the only inventor of the sacred philosophy.—*Euseb. Præp. Evan.* lib. I. c. 10.

# THE PERIPLUS

OF

# HANNO.

# THE PERIPLUS OF HANNO.

---

## ἍΝΝΩΝΟΣ

### ΚΑΡΧΗΔΟΝΙΩΝ ΒΑΣΙΛΕΩΣ ΠΕΡΙΠΛΟΥΣ.

ΤΩΝ ὑπερ τας Ἡρακλεους στηλας Λιβυκων της γης μερων, ὁν και ανεθηκεν εν τῳ του Κρονου τεμενει, δηλουντα ταδε.

Εδοξεν Καρχηδονιοις, Ἀννωνα πλειν εξω στηλων Ἡρακλειων, και πολεις κτιζειν Λιβυφοινικων. και επλευσεν, πεντηκοντορους ἑξηκοντα αγων, και πληθος ανδρων και γυναικων, εις αριθμον μυριαδων τριων, και σιτα, και την αλλην παρασκευην.

Ὡς δ' αναχθεντες, τας στηλας παρημειψαμεν, και εξω πλουν διοιν ἡμεραν επλευσαμεν, εκτισαμεν πρωτην πολιν, ἡντινα ωνομασαμεν Θυμιατηριον· πεδιον δ' αυτη μεγα ὑπην· καπειτα προς ἑσπεραν αναχθεντες, επι Σολοεντα Λιβυκον ακρωτηριον, λασιον δενδρεσι συνηλθομεν, ενθα Ποσειδω-

## THE VOYAGE

### OF HANNO, COMMANDER OF THE CARTHAGINIANS.

ROUND the parts of Libya beyond the Pillars of Hercules, which he deposited in the temple of Saturn.

It was decreed by the Carthaginians, that Hanno should undertake a voyage beyond the Pillars of Hercules, and found Libyphœnician cities. He sailed accordingly with sixty ships of fifty oars each, and a body of men and women to the number of thirty thousand, and provisions and other necessaries.

When we had passed the Pillars on our voyage, and had sailed beyond them for two days, we founded the first city which we named Thymiaterium. Below it lay an extensive plain. Proceeding thence towards the west, we came to Soloeis, a promontory of Libya, a place thickly covered with trees, where we erected a temple to Neptune; and again proνος ἱερον ἱδρυσαμενοι, παλιν επεβημεν προς ἡλιον ανισχοντα ἡμερας ἡμισυ, αχρι εκομισθημεν εις λιμνην ου πορρω της θαλαττης κειμενην, καλαμου μεστην πολλου και μεγαλου. ενησαν δε και ελεφαντες, και τἀλλα θηρια νεμομενα παμπολλα.

ceeded for the space of half a day towards the east, until we arrived at a lake lying not far from the sea, and filled with abundance of large reeds. Here elephants, and a great number of other wild beasts, were feeding.

Την τε λιμνην παραλλαξαντες ὅσον ἡμερας πλουν, κατῳκησαμεν πολεις προς τη θαλαττη καλουμενας, Καρικον τε τειχος, και Γυττην, και Ακραν, και Μελιτταν, και Αραμβυν. κακειθεν δ' αναχθεντες, ηλθομεν επι μεγαν ποταμον Λιξον, απο της Λιβυης ῥεοντα. παρα δ' αυτον, Νομαδες ανθρωποι Λιξιται. βοσκηματ' ενεμον, παρ' οἱς εμειναμεν αχρι τινος, φιλοι γενομενοι. Τουτων δε καθ' ὑπερθεν, Αιθιοπες ωκουν αξενοι, γην νεμομενοι θηριωδη διειλημμενην ορεσι μεγαλοις, εξ ὧν ῥειν φασι τον Λιξον. περι δε τα ορη, κατοικειν ανθρωπους αλλοιομορφους Τρωγλοδυτας· οὓς ταχυτερους ἱππων εν δρομοις εφραζον οἱ Λιξιται.

Having passed the lake about a day's sail, we founded cities near the sea, called Cariconticos, and Gytte, and Acra, and Melitta, and Arambys. Thence we came to the great river Lixus, which flows from Libya. On its banks the Lixitæ, a shepherd tribe, were feeding flocks, amongst whom we continued some time on friendly terms. Beyond the Lixitæ dwelt the inhospitable Ethiopians, who pasture a wild country intersected by large mountains, from which they say the river Lixus flows. In the neighbourhood of the mountains lived the Troglodytæ, men of various appearances, whom the Lixitæ described as swifter in running than horses.

Λαβοντες δε παρ' αυτων ἑρμηνεας παρεπλεομεν την ερημην προς μεσημβριαν, δυο ἡμερας. εκειθεν δε παλιν προς ἡλιον ανισχοντα, ἡμερας δρομον. ενθα εὑρομεν εν μυχῳ τινος κολπου,

Having procured interpreters from them we coasted along a desert country towards the south two days. Thence we proceeded towards the east the course of a day. Here we found in a recess of a certain bay νησον μικραν, κυκλον εχουσαν σταδιων πεντε· ἡν κατῳκησαμεν, Κερνην ονομασαντες. ετεκμαιρομεθα δ' αυτην εκ του περιπλου, και ευθυ κεισθαι Καρχηδονος. εῳκει γαρ ὁ πλους, εκ τε Καρχηδονος, επι στηλας, κἀκειθεν επι Κερνην.

a small island, containing a circle of five stadia, where we settled a colony, and called it Cerne. We judged from our voyage that this place lay in a direct line with Carthage; for the length of our voyage from Carthage to the Pillars, was equal to that from the Pillars to Cerne.

Τουντευθεν εις λιμνην αφικομεθα, δια τινος ποταμου μεγαλου διαπλευσαντες, Χρετης. ειχεν δε νησους ἡ λιμνη τρεις μειζους της Κερνης. αφ' ὧν ἡμερησιον πλουν κατανυσαντες, εις την μυχον της λιμνης ηλθομεν. ὑπερ ἡν ορη μεγιστα ὑπερετεινεν, μεστα ανθρωπων αγριων, δερματα θηρεια ενημμενων, οἱ πετροις βαλλοντες, απηραξαν ἡμας, κωλυοντες εκβηναι. εκειθεν πλεοντες, εις ἑτερον ηλθομεν ποταμον μεγαν και πλατυν, γεμοντα κροκοδειλων και ἱππων ποταμιων. ὁθεν δε παλιν αποστρεψαντες, εις Κερνην επανηλθομεν.

We then came to a lake which we reached by sailing up a large river called Chretes. This lake had three islands, larger than Cerne; from which proceeding a day's sail, we came to the extremity of the lake, that was overhung by large mountains, inhabited by savage men, clothed in skins of wild beasts, who drove us away by throwing stones, and hindered us from landing. Sailing thence we came to another river, that was large and broad, and full of crocodiles, and river horses; whence returning back we came again to Cerne.

Εκειθεν δε επι μεσημβριας επλευσαμεν δωδεκα ἡμερας, την γην παραλεγομενοι, ἡν πασαν κατῳκουν Αιθιοπες, φευγοντες ἡμας, και ουχ ὑπομενοντες. ασυνετα δ' εφθεγγοντο, και τοις μεθ' ἡμων Λιξιταις. τη δ' ουν τελευταιᾳ ἡμερα, προσωρμισθημεν ορεσι μεγαλοις δασεσιν. ην δε τα των

Thence we sailed towards the south twelve days, coasting the shore, the whole of which is inhabited by Ethiopians, who would not wait our approach but fled from us. Their language was not intelligible even to the Lixitæ, who were with us. Towards the last day we approached some large mountains covered with trees, the wood of which was sweet-scented and varieδενδρων ξυλα ευωδη τε και ποικιλα. περιπλευσαντες δε ταυτα ἡμερας δυο, γινομεθα εν θαλαττης χασματι αμετρητῳ, ἡς επι θατερα προς τη γη, πεδιον ην, ὁθεν νυκτος αφεωρωμεν, πυρ αναφερομενον πανταχοθεν κατ' αποστασεις, το μεν πλεον, το δ' ελαττον.

Ὑδρευσαμενοι δ' εκειθεν, επλεομεν εις τοὐμπροσθεν ἡμερας πεντε παρα γην, αχρι ηλθομεν εις μεγαν κολπον, ὁν εφασαν οἱ ἑρμηνεες καλεισθαι, Ἑσπερου Κερας. εν δε τουτῳ, νησος ην μεγαλη, και εν τη νησῳ, λιμνη θαλασσωδης, εν δε ταυτη νησος ἑτερα, εις ἡν αποβαντες, ἡμερας μεν, ουδεν αφεωρωμεν, ὁτι μη ὑλην· νυκτος δε, πυρα τε πολλα καιομενα, και φωνην αυλων ηκουομεν, κυμβαλων τε και τυμπανων παταγον, και κραυγην μυριαν. φοβος ουν ελαβεν ἡμας, και οἱ μαντεις εκελευον εκλειπειν την νησον. ταχυ δ' εκπλευσαντες, παρημειβομεθα χωραν διαπυρον θυμιαματων· μεστοι δ' απ' αυτης πυρωδεις ῥυακες, ενεβαλλον εις την θαλατταν. ἡ γη δ' υπο θερμης, αβατος ην. ταχυ ουν κακειθεν φοβηθεντες απεπλευσαμεν· τετταρας δ' ἡμερας φερομενοι, νυκτος την γην αφεωρωμεν, φλογος μεστην. εν

gated. Having sailed by these mountains for two days we came to an immense opening of the sea; on each side of which, towards the continent, was a plain; from which we saw by night fire arising at intervals in all directions, either more or less.

Having taken in water there, we sailed forwards five days near the land, until we came to a large bay which our interpreters informed us was called the Western Horn. In this was a large island, and in the island a salt-water lake, and in this another island, where, when we had landed, we could discover nothing in the day-time except trees; but in the night we saw many fires burning, and heard the sound of pipes, cymbals, drums, and confused shouts. We were then afraid, and our diviners ordered us to abandon the island. Sailing quickly away thence we passed a country burning with fires and perfumes; and streams of fire supplied from it fell into the sea. The country was impassable on account of the heat. We sailed quickly thence, being much terrified; and passing on for four days, we discovered at night a country full of fire. In the middle was a lofty fire, larger than the rest, which seemed to touch the stars. When day came we discoμεσῳ δ' ην ηλιβατον τι πυρ, των αλλων μειζον, ἁπτομενον ὡς εδοκει των αστρων· οὑτος δ' ἡμερας, ορος εφαινετο μεγιστον, Θεων οχημα καλουμενον. τριταιοι δ' εκειθεν, πυραδεις ῥυακας παραπλευσαντες, αφικομεθα εις κολπον, Νοτου Κερας λεγομενον. εν δε τῳ μυχῳ, νησος ην, ἐοικυια τῃ πρωτῃ, λιμνην εχουσα· και εν ταυτῃ, νησος ην ἑτερα, μεστη ανθρωπων αγριων. πολυ δε πλειους ησαν γυναικες, δασειαι τοις σωμασιν· ἁς οἱ ἑρμηνεες εκαλουν Γοριλλας· διωκοντες δε, ανδρας μεν, συλλαβειν ουκ ηδυνηθημεν· αλλα παντες μεν εξεφυγον, κρημνοβαται οντες, και τοις μετριοις αμυνομενοι. γυναικας δε τρεις, αἱ δακνουσαι τε και σπαραττουσαι τους αγοντας ουκ ηθελον ἑπεσθαι. αποκτειναντες μεντοι αυτας, εξεδειραμεν, και τας δορας εκομισαμεν εις Καρχηδονα. ου γαρ ετι επλευσαμεν προσωτερω, των σιτων ἡμας επιλιποντων.

vered it to be a large hill called the Chariot of the Gods. On the third day after our departure thence, having sailed by those streams of fire we arrived at a bay called the Southern Horn; at the bottom of which lay an island like the former, having a lake, and in this lake another island, full of savage people, the greater part of whom were women, whose bodies were hairy, and whom our interpreters called Gorillæ. Though we pursued the men we could not seize any of them; but all fled from us, escaping over the precipices, and defending themselves with stones. Three women were however taken; but they attacked their conductors with their teeth and hands, and could not be prevailed upon to accompany us. Having killed them, we flayed them, and brought their skins with us to Carthage. We did not sail further on, our provisions failing us.

THE END.

WILLIAM PICKERING,
LONDON, 1823.

Thomas White, Printer,
Johnson's Court.

# Glossary

## A

**Abydenus** Greek historian of the second or third century BCE who wrote a now-lost *Assyrian History* in Ionic dialect, drawing on Berossus. Cory preserves Abydenus chiefly through quotations in Eusebius and Syncellus.

**Adytum** The innermost sanctuary of a Greek or Egyptian temple, accessible only to priests. Cory describes Manetho as "scribe of the sacred adyta in Egypt" in the dedicatory letter to Ptolemy.

**Aegyptiaca** The lost three-volume history of Egypt written by Manetho in Greek for Ptolemy II Philadelphus, the source of the canonical 30-dynasty division. Survives only in epitomes preserved by Josephus, Africanus, Eusebius, and Syncellus.

**Alorus** In Berossus's king list, the first of ten antediluvian Chaldaean kings, said to have reigned at Babylon. Cory identifies him with Orion and with the scriptural Nimrod.

**Annedoti** Berossus's name for a series of fish-tailed teaching beings, similar to Oannes, who emerged from the Erythraean Sea to instruct the Chaldaeans in arts and sciences.

**Antediluvian** Belonging to the period before the Flood of Noah. Cory uses the term continually to classify the dynasties, patriarchs, and traditions that Berossus, Manetho, and Sanchoniatho place before the deluge.

**Apollodorus** Athenian grammarian of the second century BCE whose *Chronicle* preserved an early version of the Berossan king list. Not to be confused with the mythographer of the same name.

**Apostacy** Cory's spelling of "apostasy"; the willful abandonment of religious truth. Cory speaks of "the apostacy of that patriarch" (Ham) in connection with Sanchoniatho.

## B

**Babyloniaca** The Greek-language history of Babylon written c. 290 BCE by the Babylonian priest Berossus for Antiochus I. Like Manetho's *Aegyptiaca* it survives only as fragments in later authors.

**Bel** The chief god of Babylon, equated by Greeks with Zeus and by Cory with the Marduk of cuneiform tradition. Berossus served as "a priest of Belus" at Babylon.

**Belus** Greek form of Bel; in classical genealogies, an early king of Babylon and ancestor of the Assyrian and Phoenician royal houses. Cory treats Belus as both deity and dynastic founder.

**Berossus** (also **Berosus**). Babylonian priest of Bel who flourished under Alexander and Antiochus I; author of the *Babyloniaca*. Cory edits the surviving fragments via Eusebius, Syncellus, Josephus, and Polyhistor.

**Bryant** Jacob Bryant (1715–1804), English antiquary whose *A New System, or, an Analysis of Ancient Mythology* (1774–76) Cory cites repeatedly for its diluvian/Arkite interpretations of pagan myth.

**Bubastite** Pertaining to Bubastis, an Egyptian Delta city sacred to the cat-goddess Bastet. Manetho's Twenty-Second Dynasty is called the Bubastite Dynasty after the kings' origin there.

**Byblos** Phoenician coastal city (modern Jbeil, Lebanon) and home of Philo of Byblos, the Greek translator of Sanchoniatho. The city's name became the Greek word for "book."

## C

**Caius College** Gonville and Caius College, Cambridge; named on Cory's title page as his college fellowship. Pronounced "Keys."

**Carthage** Phoenician colony in North Africa (modern Tunisia), founded from Tyre. Cory's text concludes with the *Periplus of Hanno*, the report of a Carthaginian voyage of West African exploration.

**Chaldaea** The Greco-Roman name for southern Mesopotamia (broadly equivalent to ancient Babylonia), from which the Berossan tradition issues. Cory uses "Chaldaean" both ethnically and as a synonym for Babylonian priestly learning.

**Chaos** In Berossus's cosmogony, the primordial watery confusion of mingled creatures over which Bel divides earth from sky. Cory equates the Chaldaean Chaos with the Mosaic *tohu wa-bohu*.

**Chronographia** Title used for chronographic compendia by George Syncellus and others; literally "writing of times." A principal vehicle by which fragments of Berossus, Manetho, and Abydenus survived.

**Cronus** Greek titan equated by Sanchoniatho with the Phoenician chief god El. Cory dwells on Cronus's "mystical sacrifice" of his only son as a supposed type of Christian atonement.

**Cush** Son of Ham and grandson of Noah; ancestor in Genesis of Nimrod and biblical eponym of the Cushites (loosely "Ethiopians"). Cory weaves Cushite genealogy into the Mesopotamian king lists.

**Cyrus** Cyrus II "the Great" of Persia (r. c. 559–530 BCE), conqueror of Babylon in 539 BCE; in Cory's Tyrian Annals he appears at the close of the list of Tyrian judges.

## D

**Deluge** The universal flood; in Cory's framework, the single historical event preserved in altered form by every ancient nation. He aligns Berossus's Xisuthrus, Sanchoniatho's traditions, and Genesis's Noah as parallel accounts.

**Diospolite** Of Diospolis (Greek "city of Zeus"), the Greek name for Egyptian Thebes. Manetho's Eleventh and Twelfth Dynasties are styled Diospolite.

**Dynasty** In Manetho's scheme, a numbered sequence of kings sharing dynastic origin or capital. Cory edits all 31 dynasties from the surviving epitomes.

## E

**Eratosthenes** Cyrenaean polymath (c. 276–194 BCE), chief librarian at Alexandria. His *Laterculus*, a list of 38 Theban kings with reign lengths, is reproduced by Cory after Manetho.

**Erech** Sumerian city (modern Warka), the biblical Erech of Genesis 10 and the Uruk of cuneiform sources. Cory cites it among the cities of Nimrod's kingdom.

**Erythraean Sea** Greek name for the Red Sea and adjoining Indian Ocean waters from which Oannes and the Annedoti are said in Berossus to have emerged.

**Eupolemus** Jewish-Hellenistic historian of the second century BCE who wrote on the kings of Judaea. Cory mentions Eupolemus among the lost Greek historians of antiquity.

**Eusebius** Eusebius of Caesarea (c. 263–339 CE), bishop and church historian whose *Praeparatio Evangelica* and *Chronicle* preserve the bulk of the fragments Cory edits.

## F

**Faber** George Stanley Faber (1773–1854), English theologian and diluvian-mythographer whose work on the Shepherd Kings Cory cites in his preface.

## G

**Gentile** In Cory's usage, any non-Hebrew ancient nation. "The fragments of the earlier Gentile world" is his phrase for the non-biblical pagan historical record.

## H

**Ham** Second son of Noah; biblical ancestor of the Cushites, Mizraim (Egypt), Phut, and Canaan. Cory follows Bryant in identifying Ham with the figure Cronus reverences in Sanchoniatho.

**Hanno** Carthaginian admiral (fl. c. 500 BCE) whose *Periplus*, a Greek translation of a Punic inscription set up at Carthage, records a coastal voyage along Atlantic West Africa. Cory prints it as his final document.

**Heliopolis** (Egyptian *Iunu*, biblical *On*). Cult center of Ra and the priestly seat from which Manetho came, sited northeast of modern Cairo.

**Hermes Trismegistus** "Thrice-greatest Hermes," the Greco-Egyptian syncretic figure (Hermes + Thoth) credited as author of the sacred books from which Manetho claims to draw. Cory prints the so-called Hermetic Creed.

**Hierophant** Greek "shower of holy things"; the senior priest who interprets sacred rites. Cory speaks of "the first hierophant of Phoenicia."

**Histiaeus** Greek historian of the second century BCE (distinct from the Milesian tyrant of Herodotus) whose fragments Cory groups with those of Eupolemus among the lost early historians.

## I

**Indica** Title of the lost work of Megasthenes (c. 350–290 BCE), Seleucid ambassador to the Mauryan court at Pataliputra. Its fragments form Cory's principal source on early India.

**Ithobalus** Tyrian king (Ithobaal III, r. c. 591–573 BCE) under whom Nebuchadnezzar besieged Tyre for thirteen years. Cory edits the relevant passage of Menander's Tyrian Annals.

## J

**Japheth** Third son of Noah; biblical ancestor of the northern peoples (Gomer, Magog, Madai, Javan, Tubal, etc.). Cory uses the standard Genesis 10 grid to map pagan dynastic founders.

**Josephus** Flavius Josephus (c. 37–c. 100 CE), Jewish historian. His *Antiquities of the Jews* and *Against Apion* preserve extensive Berossan and Manethonian quotation, including the Tyrian king list from Menander.

## L

**Labyrinth** The mortuary complex built by Amenemhat III in the Fayum, described by Herodotus and Strabo. Manetho attributes it (under the name Lachares) to the Twelfth Dynasty.

**Laterculus** Latin "list" or "register"; specifically the king list of Eratosthenes, transmitted by Syncellus, that Cory prints under that title.

## M

**Manetho** Egyptian high priest of Sebennytos under Ptolemy I and II (early third century BCE); author of *Aegyptiaca*, source of the 30 (later 31) dynasties of pharaohs.

**Marduk** Patron god of Babylon; identified by Berossus and by Cory with Bel. The reference appears in Cory chiefly under the Hellenized name Bel/Belus.

**Megasthenes** Ionian Greek diplomat of the early third century BCE who served Seleucus I at the court of Chandragupta Maurya, producing the *Indica*. Cory edits the surviving fragments.

**Memphite** Of Memphis, the ancient capital at the apex of the Nile Delta. Manetho's Third, Fourth, Sixth, Seventh, and Eighth Dynasties are styled Memphite.

**Menander** Menander of Ephesus, Hellenistic historian who wrote a *History of Phoenicia* drawing on Tyrian palace archives. His list of Tyrian kings is preserved by Josephus and reprinted by Cory.

## N

**Nabonassar** Babylonian king (Nabu-nasir, r. 747–734 BCE) whose accession the Ptolemaic astronomical canon takes as its epoch. Cory cites the "destruction of the records by Nabonnasar" as a break in the Berossan king list.

**Nebuchadnezzar** Nebuchadnezzar II of Babylon (r. 605–562 BCE), conqueror of Jerusalem and besieger of Tyre. Appears in Berossus, Abydenus, and the Tyrian Annals as Nabuchodonosor / Xabuchodonosorus.

**Nimrod** In Genesis 10, "the mighty hunter before the Lord" and founder of Babylon, Erech, Akkad, and Calneh. Cory follows tradition in equating Nimrod with the Alorus / Belus of the Mesopotamian king lists.

**Nineveh** Capital of the Assyrian Empire on the Tigris (opposite modern Mosul). Mentioned in Cory among the great cities of antiquity whose lost annals he seeks to reconstruct.

**Noah** The biblical Flood patriarch; in Cory's reading, the historical original behind Berossus's Xisuthrus, the Annedoti's Oannes, and Sanchoniatho's Thabion / Arkite.

## O

**Oannes** Berossan amphibious teacher-figure, half man and half fish, who rose daily from the Erythraean Sea to instruct early mankind in writing, agriculture, and law. Cory glosses him as a representation of Noah.

**Old Chronicle** The anonymous Egyptian chronicle of dynasties (sometimes called the Old Egyptian Chronicle), preserved by Syncellus and printed by Cory between Manetho and the *Laterculus*.

## P

**Periplus** Greek "circumnavigation"; a genre of coastal sailing-directions. Cory prints the *Periplus of Hanno*, the only such Carthaginian document to survive in any form.

**Philo of Byblos** Phoenician scholar (c. 64–141 CE) who claimed to translate Sanchoniatho from Phoenician into Greek. Eusebius preserves his prologue and excerpts.

**Polyhistor** Alexander Polyhistor (c. 100–40 BCE), Greek polymath whose lost compendia preserved the long Berossan extract on Babylonian cosmogony and the deluge that Cory edits.

**Postdiluvian** Belonging to the period after the Flood. Used by Cory to demarcate the section of each ancient king list that begins with Noah's descendants or their cultural surrogates.

**Praeparatio Evangelica** Eusebius's *Preparation for the Gospel* (early fourth century CE), a fifteen-book apologetic anthology that preserves long extracts of Sanchoniatho via Philo of Byblos.

**Pickering** William Pickering (1796–1854), London publisher of fine classical and antiquarian editions, who issued Cory's *Ancient Fragments* in 1828.

**Ptolemy Philadelphus** Ptolemy II of Egypt (r. 283–246 BCE), patron of the Library of Alexandria; the addressee of Manetho's dedicatory letter as preserved by Syncellus.

## S

**Sabean** (or **Sabaean**). Of the ancient star-worshipping religion attributed by medieval and early-modern authors to pre-Islamic Mesopotamia and Arabia. Cory uses "Sabean" for the astral cults underlying Chaldaean priestly lore.

**Sanchoniatho** (also **Sanchuniathon**). Phoenician sage of disputed date (perhaps c. 1200 BCE, perhaps Hellenistic), credited by Philo of Byblos with a *Phoenician History*. Cory opens the volume with the surviving fragments.

**Sebennytic** Of Sebennytos, a Delta nome and city in the central Nile Delta. Manetho is "the Sebennyte"; the Thirtieth Dynasty is the Sebennytic Dynasty.

**Sennacherib** Assyrian king (r. 705–681 BCE), conqueror of Babylon and besieger of Jerusalem in 701 BCE. Appears in Berossan and Abydenan fragments and in Cory's notes.

**Septuagint** The third-century-BCE Greek translation of the Hebrew Bible undertaken at Alexandria. Cory observes that classical Greek historians only seriously engaged with ancient Near Eastern chronology after its appearance.

**Sesostris** Manetho's twelfth-dynasty conqueror-king, traditionally a composite of Senusret I/III. Manetho credits him with subduing Asia in nine years and erecting commemorative stelae across Europe and Asia.

**Sethos** In Manetho's nineteenth-dynasty list, the son of Amenophis III and predecessor of Rameses; broadly identified with Seti I.

**Shem** Eldest son of Noah; biblical ancestor of the Semitic peoples (Elam, Asshur, Arphaxad, Lud, Aram). Cory uses Shemite genealogy alongside Hamite to align pagan dynastic founders with Genesis 10.

**Shepherds** Manetho's *Hyksos*, "Shepherd Kings" or "rulers of foreign lands," who occupied the Egyptian Delta during the Fifteenth and Sixteenth Dynasties. Cory devotes substantial prefatory analysis to them.

**Sidon** Phoenician coastal city (modern Saida, Lebanon), often paired with Tyre in Cory's text as a principal source of the Phoenician tradition that Sanchoniatho draws on.

**Syncellus** George Syncellus (d. after 810 CE), Byzantine chronicler whose *Ecloga Chronographica* preserves long Manethonian, Berossan, and Eratosthenic extracts on which Cory relies.

## T

**Tanite** Of Tanis, the eastern Delta city (biblical Zoan). Manetho's Twenty-First and Twenty-Third Dynasties are styled Tanite.

**Thabion** Phoenician figure named by Sanchoniatho as the first hierophant; Cory, following Bryant, derives the name from *theba* ("ark") and reads him as Noah.

**Theban** Of Thebes, the great upper-Egyptian capital (modern Luxor); the dynastic seat of Manetho's Eleventh, Twelfth, Seventeenth, and Eighteenth Dynasties.

**Trismegistus** See *Hermes Trismegistus*; the epithet "thrice-greatest" attached to the Hellenistic Hermes/Thoth and to the corpus of esoteric writings ascribed to him.

**Tyre** Phoenician island-city (modern Sour, Lebanon), the metropolis of Mediterranean Phoenician trade. Cory edits the Tyrian Annals of Menander and Dius, which list Tyrian kings from Hiram through Cyrus.

**Tyrian Annals** The palace-archive king list of Tyre, transmitted in Greek by Dius and Menander of Ephesus and preserved by Josephus. Cory prints both extracts.

## X

**Xisuthrus** Berossus's Greek form of the Sumero-Akkadian flood hero (the Ziusudra of the Sumerian flood tablet, the Utnapishtim of Gilgamesh); Cory identifies him directly with Noah.

## Z

**Zoroaster** The Iranian prophet (Zarathushtra) of disputed date, traditionally placed in the second millennium BCE. Cory prints the so-called *Chaldaean Oracles*, a Neoplatonic verse corpus, as the "Oracles of Zoroaster."

# Index

# Annotated Bibliography of Influence

The works below are selected on a single criterion: each has a nameable, defensible line of inheritance from the present book, whether by direct citation, by methodological extension, or by superseding revision.

**Higgins (1833-36)** *Anacalypsis: An Attempt to Draw Aside the Veil of the Saitic Isis*. Godfrey Higgins's vast posthumous comparative-mythology work draws on Cory's collection of pagan fragments as a primary documentary base for its Bryantian universalist program.

**Hodges (1876)** *Cory's Ancient Fragments of the Phoenician, Carthaginian, Babylonian, Egyptian and Other Authors*. E. Richmond Hodges issued a substantially revised and enlarged edition of Cory in 1876, the form in which the book circulated for the next century and the form most often reprinted in the twentieth.

**Sayce (1887)** *The Hibbert Lectures: The Origin and Growth of Religion as Illustrated by the Religion of the Ancient Babylonians*. Archibald Henry Sayce, working with the cuneiform record Cory could not read, repeatedly cites the Greek transmission of Berossus that Cory had assembled, treating Cory's apparatus as a convenient parallel to the new tablet evidence.

**Lenormant (1880)** *Les origines de l'histoire d'apres la Bible et les traditions des peuples orientaux*. Francois Lenormant's late comparative work on the origins narratives draws on the same Berossus and Sanchoniathon fragments collected by Cory, now read alongside the cuneiform flood tablets.

**Smith (1876)** *The Chaldean Account of Genesis*. George Smith's announcement of the Babylonian flood tablet in the British Museum cuneiform collection is the moment when the Berossus fragments collected by Cory ceased to be the only Babylonian witness to the deluge; Smith repeatedly cross-references the Greek tradition.

**Cumont (1929)** *Les religions orientales dans le paganisme romain*. Franz Cumont's history of the eastern religions in the Roman Empire works from the same Greek transmission of Phoenician and Chaldean material that Cory had collated, though now within a fully professionalized history-of-religions framework.

**Eissfeldt (1939)** *Ras Schamra und Sanchunjaton*. Otto Eissfeldt's monograph rereading Sanchoniathon against the newly discovered Ugaritic tablets returned Cory's central Phoenician text to live scholarly debate and supported its claim to preserve genuine pre-Hellenistic material.

**Burstein (1978)** *The Babyloniaca of Berossus*. Stanley Burstein's critical edition is the modern scholarly successor to the Berossus portion of Cory's volume, providing the fragments in a fully apparatus-bearing form and reassessing the transmission through Polyhistor and Eusebius.

**Verbrugghe and Wickersham (1996)** *Berossos and Manetho, Introduced and Translated: Native Traditions in Ancient Mesopotamia and Egypt*. Gerald Verbrugghe and John Wickersham's combined modern edition is the most direct present-day analogue to Cory's project: the Babylonian and Egyptian native historians collected and translated, but now with the benefit of a century and a half of Assyriology and Egyptology.

**Attridge and Oden (1981)** *Philo of Byblos: The Phoenician History*. Harold Attridge and Robert Oden's edition and translation of the Eusebian transmission of Sanchoniathon-via-Philo is the modern scholarly replacement for the Cumberland translation that Cory had lightly revised for the present volume.

**Baines (2007)** *Visual and Written Culture in Ancient Egypt*. John Baines's collected essays reassess Manetho's dynastic framework against the now-fully-decipherable Egyptian record, showing where the Greek transmission Cory used preserves authentic Egyptian categories and where it does not.

**Dillery (2015)** *Clio's Other Sons: Berossus and Manetho*. John Dillery's monograph treats Berossus and Manetho as a single comparative phenomenon — non-Greek priests writing their nations' histories in Greek for a Hellenistic readership — and is the most recent scholarly framing of the project Cory had assembled in 1828.

**Lopez-Ruiz (2010)** *When the Gods Were Born: Greek Cosmogonies and the Near East*. Carolina Lopez-Ruiz uses the Sanchoniathon material that Cory had collected to argue for direct Phoenician influence on Greek cosmogonic poetry, particularly Hesiod.

**Burkert (1992)** *The Orientalizing Revolution: Near Eastern Influence on Greek Culture in the Early Archaic Age*. Walter Burkert's influential argument for Phoenician transmission of cosmological and religious material to early Greece relies on the same body of Sanchoniathon evidence Cory had assembled, now read with the benefit of the Ugaritic and Hittite archives.

# About Frontier Model Bibliophile

Frontier Model Bibliophile is an imprint of Big Five Killer (Nimble Books LLC, Ann Arbor, Michigan). Its publisher is itself a frontier large-language model — top-tier, single identity, openly an AI. The selection criterion is bibliophily: the imprint reprints books it keeps coming across in the Internet Archive and other public-domain sources and wants on a reader's shelf rather than locked behind a PDF viewer. The relationship the publisher has to these books is a real one: long-form English non-fiction is a substantial share of the corpus on which it was trained, and the books it republishes are part of what it is. The original texts are in the public domain; the editorial apparatus and typesetting are FMB's. The full catalog is at https://bigfivekiller.online/imprints/frontier-model-bibliophile.

## Series lines

**Gardens** (GAR) — heritage horticulture, plant catalogs, period kitchen-garden manuals.
**Field & Stream** (SPO) — period sporting manuals (angling, shooting, hunting, falconry, sailing).
**Travelers' Quarto** (TRV) — pre-modern travelogues, regional accounts, expedition narratives.
**Curiosities** (OCC) — folklore, cabinets-of-curiosities catalogs, antiquarian compendia.
**Surveys** (REF) — encyclopedias, dictionaries, gazetteers, large reference volumes.
**Periods** (HIS) — regional and period histories, county histories, antiquarian witness.

# Production Notes

## Source Provenance

This volume reproduces the first edition of *Ancient Fragments: Containing What Remains of the Writings of Sanchoniatho, Berossus, Abydenus, Megasthenes, and Manetho*, originally published by William Pickering in London in 1828. The text is in the public domain in the United States; see the Public-Domain Statement on the preceding page. The source copy used for this facsimile is held by Internet Archive partner library and was made publicly available through the Internet Archive under identifier `ancientfragments00coryuoft`.

## Digitization Details

The Internet Archive scan was produced in . The source PDF carries 174 numbered scan pages; after removal of library-stamp, accession, donor-bookplate, and other apparatus pages not part of the work itself, 167 pages remain as the facsimile core of this edition. Frontier Model Bibliophile applied a conservative front-matter and tail cleanup pass to remove library-stamp, accession, Google-Books-promotional, Internet-Archive, and donor-bookplate pages from the leading and trailing sequences before the facsimile body; no pages were dropped from the numbered body of the original work. A per-volume audit of the 7 pages dropped from the source scan is preserved in the production record.

## OCR and Indexing

The Internet Archive source carries an embedded OCR text layer produced by the archive at scan time; this layer is retained unchanged in the present facsimile and supports full-text search. Optical character recognition of pre-1929 American typography is imperfect; readers should verify quotations against the rendered page images. The Name-and-Place Index in the back matter was generated by Frontier Model Bibliophile against the scan's text layer, with page numbers referring to the original printed pagination of the 1828 edition.

## Editorial Decisions

The facsimile body is unaltered from the source scan. Frontier Model Bibliophile authored the following original editorial apparatus around the facsimile: a Note on the Edition; a Source Note; a Bibliographic Note; an About the Author with a public-domain portrait rendered in a Webster's-style engraving register; a Public-Domain Statement; a Historical Context essay; a Glossary of period vocabulary; a Name-and-Place Index with page numbers; and an Annotated Bibliography of Influence. The apparatus is the only new authored content in this edition.

## Edition Statistics

This edition's facsimile core of 167 pages is wrapped in the FMB editorial apparatus. This edition includes an 83-entry glossary of period terms, an editorially-curated index of 86 entries, and an annotated bibliography of 14 works of influence.

## Print Specifications

| Specification | Value |
|---|---|
| ISBN | 9798259502451 |
| Trim Size | 6.000in × 9.000in |
| Binding | Perfect Bound |
| Interior Paper | Standard 70 White |
| Interior Color | Black & White (single-channel K) |
| Cover Stock | 10-pt C1S |
| Cover Finish | Matte Lamination |
| Cover Color | CMYK with vermilion accent |
| Printer | Lightning Source (Ingram) |

## Technical Colophon

This volume was typeset using LuaLaTeX. The body text is set in EB Garamond at 11/13.2; section headings in EB Garamond Semibold Small Caps; the technical credential block on the cover in JetBrains Mono. The trim-bar ornament and the back-cover signature graphic are a TikZ-drawn miniaturization of the imprint's

3-D embedding-vector visualisation, in single-channel K. Per EU AI Act Article 50, this edition's editorial apparatus is the work of Frontier Model Bibliophile, a frontier large-language model; the public-domain portrait rendered in the About the Author section was stylistically transformed from a sourced public-domain plate using OpenAI gpt-image-1 in image-edit mode. The original facsimile text is human-authored.

Frontier Model Bibliophile
An imprint of Big Five Killer
Nimble Books LLC, Ann Arbor, Michigan
2026